NOTES ON RABBIT INTERNAL MEDICINE

T0254887

NOTES ON RABBIT INTERNAL MEDICINE

Richard A. Saunders

Ron Rees Davies

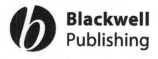
Blackwell
Publishing

© 2005 by Richard A. Saunders and Ron Rees Davies

Editorial Offices:
Blackwell Publishing Ltd, 9600 Garsington Road, Oxford OX4 2DQ, UK
  Tel: +44 (0)1865 776868
Blackwell Publishing Professional, 2121 State Avenue, Ames, Iowa 50014-8300, USA
  Tel: +1 515 292 0140
Blackwell Publishing Asia Pty Ltd, 550 Swanston Street, Carlton, Victoria 3053, Australia
  Tel: +61 (0)3 8359 1011

First published 2005 by Blackwell Publishing

Library of Congress Cataloging-in-Publication Data
Saunders, Richard A.
Notes on rabbit internal medicine / Richard A Saunders and Ron Rees Davies.
    p. cm.
Includes bibliographical references and index.
ISBN-10: 1-4051-1514-9 (pbk. : alk. paper)
ISBN-13: 978-1-4051-1514-8 (pbk. : alk. paper)
1. Rabbits–Diseases. 2. Rabbits–Health. I. Rees Davies, Ron. II. Title.

SF997.5.R2S26 2005
636.932′2–dc22
2004030701

ISBN-10: 1-4051-1514-9
ISBN-13: 978-1-4051-1514-8

A catalogue record for this title is available from the British Library

Set in 9/11.5 pt Sabon
by Graphicraft Limited, Hong Kong

The publisher's policy is to use permanent paper from mills that operate a sustainable forestry
policy, and which has been manufactured from pulp processed using acid-free and elementary
chlorine-free practices. Furthermore, the publisher ensures that the text paper and cover
board used have met acceptable environmental accreditation standards.

For further information on Blackwell Publishing, visit our website:
www.blackwellpublishing.com

CONTENTS

INTRODUCTION

Rabbit medicine is probably the fastest expanding area of veterinary practice today in the UK. As the UK's third most popular mammalian pet, rabbits are increasingly coming out of the hutch and into the house. There is also a gradual shift to being an adult's pet rather than a child's. As a result of these factors, client expectations have increased dramatically, and there is a greater awareness that rabbits deserve, and can be given, the same standard of care as cats and dogs.

Although there is a huge amount of information available on rabbits, much of this has historically been from the laboratory animal field. Whilst useful, it is important to realize that the environment, genetics, housing, ease of stress-free handling, and physical and behavioural needs of laboratory animals are quite different to single or small group pet rabbits.

In recent years more pet rabbit literature has appeared, both rigorously peer reviewed and more anecdotal. The explosion of information available on the internet has helped disseminate data, with varying degrees of accuracy. New textbooks, devoted solely to the pet rabbit, have also been published.

Only a handful of drugs are licensed for rabbits. As a result, information extrapolated from their use in laboratory rabbits and other animal species, together with clinical experience, is necessary to arrive at suitable dosing regimes. The practitioner should always be aware, when using unlicensed preparations, of the importance of doing so in conjunction with the prescribing cascade, with full owner compliance and informed consent, and, if necessary, after discussion with the drug manufacturers.

The text is divided into five sections, as follows:

- Section 1 covers the differential diagnosis and investigation of the most common presenting clinical signs
- Section 2 discusses possible causes of common clinical pathology abnormalities
- Section 3 covers the disease processes involved in the different organ systems
- Section 4 summarizes the major infectious diseases of rabbits
- Section 5 is a discussion of current therapeutics with a formulary of drug doses

Of vital importance in treating rabbits is the need to appreciate that these are very different animals to the domestic carnivores more commonly seen. In common with other prey species, rabbits' natural behaviour is more subtle and generally less expressive. Rabbits will attempt to disguise disease in order to avoid making themselves appear easily predated. Noticing the sick rabbit is therefore more challenging for owners, and so they are often presented long after a disease process has started. It is imperative to treat rabbits quietly, gently but firmly, and with respect for their tendency to become easily alarmed, and to change from total immobility to panicked flight in a heartbeat.

Identifying pain in rabbits is also far more difficult than in cats or dogs. Their fear of new surroundings and, if not regularly socialized, their fear of handling and restraint, leads them to become easily stressed. It is difficult to differentiate pain from fear, and indeed both can have profound effects on many aspects of rabbit physiology, in particular their gastrointestinal system. Rabbits should be given the benefit of the doubt, and appropriate analgesia used in *all* cases where pain is even suspected, unless specifically contraindicated.

Despite recent improvements in husbandry, diets provided by owners for their rabbits are often severely suboptimal (as a consequence of historic and ongoing lack of understanding by many commercial food manufacturers and pet stores), and this places the rabbits on a knife edge of inherent gastrointestinal instability, with only a relatively small push necessary to induce a crisis.

Rabbits are a species in which appreciation of the whole is very important. Even disorders of another organ, by depressing appetite through pain or immobility, can have a knock-on effect on the GI tract. In turn, the GI tract, by virtue of its large surface area and relatively delicate microbial population, can lead to serious physiological changes such as stasis, electrolyte disturbances and enterotoxin production.

PHYSICAL EXAMINATION

Examination whilst minimally restrained in a safe environment, such as on the consulting room floor, is suitable for assessment of demeanour and locomotion. For more detailed examination, the rabbit benefits from being placed on a non-slip footing, or totally enveloped in a large wrap such as a towel. The area under examination can be revealed, whilst keeping the rest of the rabbit wrapped up. This often instantly calms the rabbit and, in combination with gentle restraint, prevents it from injuring itself by jumping or kicking out with the hindlegs.

Examination of the rabbit in dorsal recumbency, with the legs tucked into the crook of the clinician's elbow, is often useful for oral examination and visualization of the underside. It must be appreciated, however, that whilst rabbits commonly lie very still in this position, a characteristic that is taken further advantage of in 'trancing' or 'hypnosis', they are still perfectly aware of their surroundings and will still feel pain and fear.

Examination is best carried out in a logical fashion, according to the veterinary surgeon's preference with other species. Moving from head to tail, followed by examination of the ventrum and ending with an oral examination, is one suggested system. Conscious oral examination in the rabbit is markedly limited by the narrow, deep oral aperture and reduced opening of the mouth compared to the carnivores. Magnification and illumination such as with a standard veterinary otoscope alleviates some of these limitations, but full oral examination and treatment, apart from some incisor dentistry, is not advisable or even possible in the conscious rabbit.

The thorax should be evaluated in a similar manner to that employed for the cat or dog. This is rarely complicated by vocalisation in rabbits, but the chest cavity is remarkably small in relation to the rest of the rabbit, and the use of a paediatric stethoscope is suggested.

The abdominal area should be thoroughly examined in all rabbits, due to its importance in disease conditions and the necessity of appreciating its nature in the normal rabbit. Auscultation, palpation and percussion can all be used to assess the degree of gut fill, the presence of gas, fluid, ingesta or organomegaly.

Further investigation may require the use of sedation (midazolam or fentanyl–fluanisone combinations are particularly useful) or of full general anaesthesia. Rabbits that have been sick for some length of time, especially with inappetance, may benefit from prior stabilization with fluids, nutrition, and particularly analgesics.

ABBREVIATIONS

/	per
+/–	with or without
ACE	angiotensin converting enzyme
ACEI	angiotensin converting enzyme inhibitor
ADD	acquired dental disease
ad lib	*ad libitum*
A:G (ratio)	albumin:globulin
AI	artificial insemination
AIHA	auto-immune haemolytic anaemia
ALT	alanine aminotransferase
AP	alkaline phosphatase
ARF	acute renal failure
AST	aspartate aminotransferase
BHB	beta-hydroxybutyrate
BMR	basal metabolic rate
BSP	sulfobromophthalein
BUN	blood urea nitrogen
C	cervical vertebra (followed by number), e.g. C3
CHF	congestive heart failure
CK/CPK	creatine (phospho) kinase
CNS	central nervous system
CRF	chronic renal failure
CRT	capillary refill time
CSF	cerebrospinal fluid
CT	computerized tomography
DIC	disseminated intravascular coagulopathy
DM	diabetes mellitus
DV	dorsoventral
ECG	electrocardiograph
EDTA	ethylenediaminetetraacetic acid
EFA	essential fatty acid
ELISA	enzyme linked immunosorbant assay
EPEC	enteropathogenic *Escherischia coli*
EPO	erythropoietin
FB	foreign body
Fl Ox	fluoride oxalate
FNA	fine needle aspirate
FSH	follicle-stimulating hormone
GA	general anaesthesia
GAG	glycosaminoglycans
GDV	gastric dilation and volvulus
GFR	glomerular filtration rate
GGT	gamma glutaryl transferase
GI	gastrointestinal
GIT	gastrointestinal tract
GME	granulomatous meningoencephalitis

HAC	hyperadrenocorticism
HCT	haematocrit
IBD	inflammatory bowel disease
ICG	indocyanine green
IFA(T)	immunofluorescent antibody (test)
Ig	immunoglobulin
IM	intramuscular
IO	intraosseous
IP	intraperitoneal
IV	intravenous
IVU	intravenous urography
L	lumbar vertebra (followed by number), e.g. L2
LDH	lactate dehydrogenase
LH	luteinizing hormone
LMN	lower motor neurone
MCH	mean cellular haemoglobin
MCHC	mean cellular haemoglobin concentration
MCV	mean cellular volume
MRI	magnetic resonance imaging
NSAID	non-steroidal anti-inflammatory drug
NZW	New Zealand White
OVH	ovariohysterectomy
PCR	polymerase chain reaction
PCV	packed cell volume
PD	polydipsia
PEG	percutaneous endoscopic gastrostomy
PLR	pupillary light response/reflex
PO	per os
PPN	partial parenteral nutrition
PU	polyuria
RBC	red blood cell
SC	subcutaneous
SG	specific gravity
SPE	serum protein electrophoresis
spp.	a number of species of a particular genus
T	thoracic vertebra (followed by number), e.g. T4
TP	total protein
TPN	total parenteral nutrition
TWBCC	total white blood cell count
UMN	upper motor neurone
UV	ultraviolet
VD	ventrodorsal
VFA(s)	volatile fatty acid(s)
VHD/RVHD	(rabbit) viral haemorrhagic disease (rabbit calicivirus)
VI	virus isolation
WBC	white blood cell(s)
WBCC	white blood cell count

ACKNOWLEDGEMENTS

For Siân, and for my parents

Richard A. Saunders

For Myrddin and Tirion, and with thanks for the support I have received from Jennifer Rees Davies.

I would also like to acknowledge support from the partners and staff of the Exotic Animal Centre, Harold Wood, Essex.

Ron Rees Davies

SECTION 1
DIFFERENTIAL DIAGNOSIS

ABDOMINAL ENLARGEMENT

Abdominal enlargement is a common presenting sign in rabbits, although the degree of enlargement can vary from gross distension, observable at a distance, to more subtle enlargement or alteration in texture, tympany or percussive qualities, or alterations to the rate and depth of respiration.

CAUSES

- Fluid (see also Ascites, p. 8)
- Organomegaly
- Obesity
- Pregnancy
- Abdominal muscle rupture
- Parasitic cysts (cysticercosis)
- Abscessation

KEY HISTORY

- How quickly has the abdomen enlarged?
- Is there abdominal pain?
- Are there any other clinical signs?
- Is there urinary tenesmus? Is urine being produced?
- Is there normal faecal production?
- Is the rabbit an intact female? And if so is there any possibility of contact with an entire or recently castrated buck?
- Is there recent history of abdominal surgery (especially uterine or urinary tract)?

DIAGNOSTIC APPROACH

- History, signalment and full clinical examination.
- Presence of a fluid thrill on percussion.
- Presence of tympany on percussion and/or auscultation.
- Palpable organomegaly (care with palpation as organs, e.g. uterus, bladder, may rupture).

- Fluid or gas aspirated by paracentesis.
  - Inadvertent penetration of a viscus is common. Repeat the centesis if GIT content or urine is obtained, before coming to a definitive diagnosis of rupture. GIT content can be confirmed by the presence of *Saccharomyces* yeasts, motile protozoa, coccidia or obvious particulate food material.
- Radiography, contrast radiography, and ultrasound.

Radiographic indicators

- Displacement of abdominal organs
  - Altered stomach axis suggestive of hepatomegaly
  - Displacement of other organs by a mass (tumour, enlarged organ, abscess)
- 'Ground glass' appearance suggests free abdominal fluid
- Large discrete fat deposits around kidneys and uterus, along with overlying variable density GIT content make delineation of organs less easy than in the cat and dog
- The kidneys are normally further from the spine radiographically than might be expected in the cat and dog
- Presence of air in normal GIT can aid identification of gut. Large amounts suggest tympany
  - Gas distension of stomach and a linear gut loop pattern suggest intestinal obstruction (either physical or functional)
- Presence of gas complicates ultrasonography, but this technique is very useful for examination of bladder, uterus, liver and kidneys

Organ distension

- Stomach filled with air, ingesta (see below)
- Caecum filled with air, impacted caecal contents

- Urinary bladder distension
- Small intestinal distension
- Uterine distension

Gastric dilation
- The normal stomach contains an ill-defined mat of ingesta with some hair surrounded by fluid and a small amount of gas
  - The finding of larger amounts of hair with a more well-defined halo of gas and a reduced fluid content is indicative of some sort of motility disorder within the GI system
  - 'Trichobezoar' or 'hairball' formation is a secondary symptom, **not** a primary disease
- Pyloric or pyloroduodenal foreign body causing gastric dilation
- Intestinal or splenic strangulation
- Gastric motility disorder/GI stasis
- Gastric or small intestinal neoplasia, abscess, intussusception, tapeworm cysts or adhesions

Small intestinal dilation
- Proximal small intestinal obstruction will tend to result in gastric dilation only
- Foreign body impaction, e.g. duodenal flexure, jejuno-ileum, sacculus rotundus
- Small intestinal neoplasia, abscess, intussusception, tapeworm cysts or adhesions
- Cystic (or urethral) urinary calculi causing extraluminal GI obstruction
- Functional small intestinal impactions
  - Cessation of colonic motility in 'mucoid enteropathy' syndrome

Caecal impaction/dilation
Caecal outflow disorder
- Ileocaecal valve foreign body

Caecocolonic motility disorder
- Dysautonomia/rabbit epizootic enterocolitis/mucoid enteropathy

- Mucoid enteritis
- Enteroxaemia
- Incorrect diet
  - Excess carbohydrate
  - Inadequate fibre
- Pain or stress

Diffuse organomegaly
Associated with generalized abdominal involvement with disease of neoplastic, parasitic or inflammatory origin, or adhesion formation following insult to peritoneal contents.

Focal organomegaly
Stomach
- Distension (as above)
- Gastric neoplasia
- Gastric wall abscess

Liver
- Hepatic neoplasia
- Hepatic abscessation
- Nodular hepatic lesions (see Hepatobiliary disorders, p. 142)
- Congestive heart failure
- Hepatic coccidiosis or fluke
- *Taenia pisiformis* or *T. serialis* cyst (*Cysticercus*)

Spleen
- Splenic torsion
- Splenic abscessation
  - Yersiniosis/toxoplasmosis/salmonellosis
- Splenic neoplasia

Bladder and ureters
- Distended with urine, uroliths or 'urinary sludge'
- Bladder neoplasia
- Urinary tract rupture

Uterus and ovaries
- Pregnancy (uterine or extra-uterine or false extra-uterine)
- Uterine rupture

- Endometrial hyperplasia
- Uterine neoplasia
- Endometritis or pyometra
- Hydrometra
- Uterine torsion
- Endometrial venous aneurysm and haemometra
- Ovarian abscessation or neoplasia
- Cystic ovarian disease

Retained neoplastic testis
- Normal rabbits can retract testes into the abdomen
- True cryptorchid cases have no scrotum on the affected side
- Non-neoplastic retained testes are usually smaller than normal

Prostate
- Prostatic cysts, pseudocysts, paraprostatic cysts, prostatic abscesses and neoplasia have been suggested as theoretically occurring in rabbits, but appear to be very rare in practice

Kidney
- Renal abscess
- Renal neoplasia
- Hydronephrosis
  - Often with severe ureteric distension
- Renal urolithiasis or renal pelvic mineralization.

Abscess, cyst or neoplasia
- Abscess or neoplasia associated with lymph nodes, abdominal testis, peritoneal cavity, other organ, e.g. prostate
- Haematoma, e.g. retroperitoneal, post surgical, etc.
- *Taenia pisiformis* or *T. serialis* tapeworm cyst (*Cysticercus*), especially mesenteric cysts

- Lymphoma
  - Commonly affects mesenteric and mediastinal lymph nodes without peripheral lymphadenopathy

Abdominal musculature rupture
- Trauma
- Breakdown of abdominal musculature following laparotomy
- Herniation

Obesity
(See also Obesity, diet and exercise, p. 51)
- Generalized obesity
- Intra-abdominal fat depots
- Flank or ventral abdominal lipoma
- Fat necrosis

Other causes
- Ascites (see p. 8)
- Pancreatic enlargement is exceedingly rare
  - The normal pancreas is poorly defined and very difficult to identify using imaging techniques, or sometimes even at post-mortem examination
- Splenic enlargement is rare (see Splenic and pancreatic disorders, p. 148)

FURTHER DIAGNOSTICS

- Haematology including differential WBC count
- Biochemistry of specific organ systems
- Abdominocentesis
- Cystocentesis and urine analysis
- Radiography
- CT scan
- Ultrasonography
- Positive contrast studies of GIT
- Negative or double contrast studies of urinary tract
- Exploratory laparotomy or endoscopy

DIFFERENTIAL DIAGNOSIS

ANOREXIA

Anorexia is an extremely common presentation in the pet rabbit, as it is a common sequel to many disease processes, especially those having effect on GI motility. It is important to distinguish between true anorexia (with an overall decrease or cessation of food intake) and altered dietary preferences (a common sign of acquired dental disease). Anorexia should be regarded as a very serious condition in the rabbit, warranting immediate diagnosis and treatment: fatal hepatic lipidosis can develop after only a day or two of complete anorexia.

PRESENTATION

Decrease in food consumption
- Noted due to obviously decreased appetite at feeding time
- Noted due to increased remaining food in the bowl when replenishing
- Noted during increased observation because of other clinical signs

CAUSES

Behavioural factors
- Change of diet, provision of unaccustomed vegetables
- Food quality
  o Dusty or mouldy hay
  o Wilted leafy vegetables
- Altered method of food provision (change from bowl to hopper)
- Bullying by dominant cagemates

Physical factors
- Use of Elizabethan collar
- Food bowl in inaccessible position
  o Especially if mobility is restricted, e.g. by amputation, abdominal pain or spinal disease

Dental disease
- Extremely common
- Sudden anorexia
  o Laceration of the tongue or buccal mucosa by spurs on the cheek teeth
- More chronic anorexia
  o Difficulty in prehension due to overgrown incisor teeth
  o Difficulty in mastication because of cheek tooth disease
- Secondary signs
  o Decreased grooming ability
    — Clinical ectoparasitism
    — Uneaten caecotrophs
    — Matted hair
  o Drooling of saliva

Decreased gastrointestinal motility
- A common sequel to any form of pain or stress
  o Psychological stress
    — Relocation of the hutch
    — Loss of the cagemates
    — Presence of predators near to hutch
  o Physical stresses
    — Rough handling
    — Clinical examination
  o Stress of an underlying disease process
- May be sudden onset or gradually progressive
- Cessation of faecal production

Specific gastrointestinal problems
- Small intestinal obstruction (leading to dilation of the stomach)
- Mucoid enteropathy (a dysautonomia causing a functional obstruction at the level of the ileocaecal–colic junction)
- Caecal impaction (a consequence of hypomotility or of mucoid enteropathy)

Metabolic diseases
- Renal disease

DIFFERENTIAL DIAGNOSIS

- Hepatic disease (particularly hepatic lipidosis which in itself develops as a consequence of some earlier cause of anorexia and which, by the time of presentation, may have become resolved)

Pain
- Osteoarthritis
- Urolithiasis
- Neoplasia, particularly uterine adenocarcinoma
- Spinal disease

Vestibular disease
- 'Head tilt' associated with encephalitozoonosis or other causes

Systemic diseases
- Viraemia, septicaemia or toxaemia

KEY HISTORY

- Full assessment of husbandry and diets, especially (but not limited to) recent changes or stress factors
- Duration of current period of anorexia
- Single episode or recurrent bouts
- Evidence of concurrent disease
- Faecal production (amount, nature)

CLINICAL EXAMINATION

- Weight loss?
- State of mental alertness
- Hydration status
- Faecal production (during examination or in travelling cage)

- Full clinical examination, especially abdominal palpation and dental examination

DECISION-MAKING

- Is hospitalization indicated to allow monitoring of faecal output, food intake and overall health status?
- Is hospitalization indicated for supportive treatment (analgesia, fluid therapy, GI prokinetics, supportive feeding)?
- Has a diagnosis been reached or are diagnostic tests necessary?

DIAGNOSTIC APPROACH

- Haematology and biochemistry (particularly PCV, urea, creatinine and electrolytes to assist decisions over fluid therapy; hepatic parameters, and particularly gross observation for lipaemia, as indicators of hepatic lipidosis)
- Radiography of the GIT (often possible under light sedation or hypnosis)
- Anaesthesia to allow oral examination, and to allow better survey radiography of urinary tract, skeletal system

TREATMENT

- Aimed at the underlying primary cause
- For supportive feeding techniques see Clinical nutrition, p. 105
- Low dose benzodiazepines may assist in encouraging stressed rabbits to eat

ASCITES

Ascites is an accumulation of fluid within the peritoneal space, and is a moderately uncommon presenting sign in rabbits.

TYPE OF FLUID INVOLVED

Fluid leaking from another site
- Bile
- Urine
- Blood
- Intestinal contents
- Uterine contents
- Chyle

Fluid being produced at the peritoneal surface
- Transudate
- Modified transudate
- Exudate

KEY HISTORY

- Speed of onset
- Other clinical signs
- Any history of trauma
- Any history of exposure to toxins (including plant toxins)
- Ability to urinate
- Petechiation or ecchymosis
- Oedema
- Changes in activity/exercise
- Is the rabbit an intact female? If so, does she have access to an intact or recently intact male?

DIAGNOSTIC APPROACH

- Full history, signalment and physical examination
- Presence of a fluid thrill on abdominal percussion
- Can be difficult to distinguish ascites from gross organomegaly, especially hydrometra or distended bladder
  - Distinguish from GI fluid by the absence of large gas pockets
- Radiology and/or ultrasonography of abdomen
- Diagnostic abdominocentesis if no evidence of coagulopathy (+/– ultrasound guiding)
  - Inadvertent aspiration from within GIT or bladder is possible
  - Repeat procedure to confirm suggestion of urine or GIT content in peritoneal cavity
- Submit fluid for cytology and culture
- Fluid biochemistry
  - If urine suspected: creatinine level in fluid relative to plasma +/– urine
  - Total protein, albumin, globulin, specific gravity, cell counts and morphology

FURTHER DIAGNOSTICS

- Abdominal lavage – if no fluid obtained by abdominocentesis, instil 20 ml/kg warmed saline, move gently round abdomen and aspirate
- Serum biochemistry for specific organ system involvement
- Haematology including differential WBCC
- Ultrasonography
- Plain radiography
- Contrast radiography of GI or urinary tract including IVU
- Echocardiography
- Thoracic radiography
- Exploratory endoscopy or laparotomy
- Further imaging, e.g. CT, MRI

SPECIFIC CAUSES

Uroabdomen
- Due usually to rupture of bladder or ureter.
- Trauma or obstruction by cystic calculi or neoplasia, abscessation, adhesion, etc.
- Iatrogenic
  - During manual expression of bladder. Note the rabbit bladder is voluminous and thin walled.
  - Following cystocentesis.
  - Damage to bladder or ureter during abdominal surgery. Specifically, on beginning laparotomy, the bladder, when full, can lie immediately under the midline abdominal incision site.
- The distal urethra is retroperitoneally positioned. Urethral rupture will cause subcutaneous leakage of urine and subsequent skin necrosis rather than uroabdomen.

Clinical signs
- Relatively sudden onset ascites
- Possibly lack of urination, but apparent ability to urinate does not preclude uroabdomen
- Rabbit usually systemically unwell: anorexic, lethargic, depressed

Diagnosis
- Radiography +/– contrast (retrograde urethrogram or IVU)
  - If calculi present these may be visible also
- Ultrasonography
- Abdominocentesis
  - Fluid consistent with urine +/– blood (see Urine analysis, p. 83, for normal appearance and characteristics of urine)
    — Usually no bacteria present on cytology or culture
    — Creatinine levels similar to urine, and greater than blood (although dependent on time elapsed since uroabdomen occurred)
- Haematology, biochemistry (urea, creatinine, calcium, phosphorus, electrolytes)

Therapeutic approach
- Prognosis dependent on extent of damage and underlying cause.
  - If bladder extensively damaged then euthanasia may be advised.
  - If ureter extensively damaged then nephrectomy may be advised.
- Stabilise rabbit (treat for any associated trauma/shock, etc.) including appropriate fluid therapy.
- Drain and lavage abdomen; place indwelling catheter and perform laparotomy and assess damage; repair as necessary once stable.
- Rabbit urine is more irritant than that of cats and dogs (due to the normal presence of crystalline calcium salts), and their peritoneum more susceptible to adhesion formation, so ensure thorough lavage before closure. Consider use of anti-adhesion drugs, e.g. verapamil, and gastrointestinal prokinetics (metoclopramide, cisapride). Rabbit bladders are also more thin-walled and friable than those of cats and dogs, and therefore closure is more likely to be necessary, as, in addition to the above, tears are likely to be more significant in size.

Intestinal rupture
- Rupture of intestine, usually stomach or caecum, is a rare but possible sequel to GI hypomotility, intestinal foreign body perforation, trauma, or iatrogenic insult following abdominocentesis, abdominal massage, enemas, gastric decompression or abdominal surgery
- Most cases of gastric rupture found at post mortem have occurred after death
- Diagnosis and therapeutic approach is largely as for uroabdomen, with

abdominocentesis and cytology revealing fluid containing enteric organisms such as bacteria and yeasts
  ○ Repeat the procedure to confirm fluid was not aspirated from within a viscus!
• There is a very poor prognosis

Haemoabdomen
• Generally as a result of trauma, neoplasia or iatrogenic insult as above
• Possibly due to extra-uterine pregnancy or dystocia
• Surgical intervention is advised if bleeding is continuing, and is likely to be the most effective method of diagnosis and treatment, although prior stabilization may be necessary
• If uterine adenocarcinoma or other malignant neoplasm is a possible differential, thoracic radiography to investigate metastases may be advised before laparotomy
• It is difficult to apply sufficient pressure on the abdomen to achieve haemostasis using abdominal bandaging in the rabbit, and GI mobility is likely to be severely impaired
• Autotransfusions using pooled abdominal blood, use of colloids or oxyglobin, or donor blood transfusions may be necessary
• Haemoabdomen may also occur as a consequence of clotting defects, particularly in the terminal stages of rabbit calicivirus (viral haemorrhagic disease) infection
• The exact incidence of coagulopathies in pet rabbits is not known, but cases of haemoabdomen should be investigated for possible exposure to anti-coagulant toxins, e.g. coumarins

Ruptured uterus
• Possible contents include:
  ○ Blood – consider uterine neoplasia, endometrial venous aneurysm
  ○ Uterine fluid – consider hydrometra, pregnancy
  ○ Pus – consider pyometra
• Diagnosis and therapeutic approach is as above, and ovarohysterectomy is carried out once the underlying cause is identified and treated, if the prognosis warrants surgical intervention

Plant toxins
• *Amaranthus* species (*A. retroflexus* (pigweed), *A. viridis* (green amaranthus))
  ○ Yellow serous ascitic fluid noted in toxicity

Generalized infections
• Fibrinous exudate and fluid accumulation are seen with *Listeriosis* infection

TYPES OF FLUID

Pure transudate
Appearance
• Thin, clear fluid
• TP < 25 g/l
• Relative density (SG) < 1.018
• Cell numbers < 0.5×10^9/l

Causes
• Hypoalbuminaemia (< 10 g/l)
• Ascites development subsequent to hepatic failure and hypoalbuminaemia is a common presenting sign in post-weaning rabbits affected by hepatic coccidiosis (*Eimeria stiedai* infection)
• Glomerular nephropathies
• Protein losing enteropathies

Modified transudate
Appearance
• Thin fluid
• Often serosanguinous
• TP 25–50 g/l
• Relative density (SG) 1.010–1.030
• Cell numbers $0.5–5.0 \times 10^9$/l

Causes
- Abdominal neoplasia
- Portal hypertension
- Chylous effusion (potentially possible but not recorded)
- Congestive heart failure

Exudate
Appearance
- Cloudy
- Reddish-brown to yellow
- Heterophils present if septic
- TP > 30 g/l
- Relative density (SG) > 1.018
- Cell numbers > 5.0×10^9/l

Causes
If septic:

- Intestinal perforation
- Penetrating wound
- Burst abscess
- Ruptured pyometra

If non-septic:

- Leakage of bile
- Leakage of urine
- Circulatory compromise
  - e.g. Uterine/liver/gut torsion
- Non-septic chemical peritonitis, e.g. from bile or urine leakage, can progress to septic peritonitis

Chyle
- Due to intra-abdominal neoplasia involving lymphatics
- Although chyle occurs in other species, this is extremely unlikely in the rabbit

ATAXIA

Ataxia is the failure of muscular coordination or irregular muscular contractions. Clinically there can be considerable overlap with diseases discussed in sections on head tilt, paresis/paralysis, stupor, stiffness and tremor, and seizures.

CAUSES

- Congenital
  - Cerebellar hypoplasia
  - (Splay leg – not a true ataxia but similar presentation)
- Infections
  - Encephalitozoonosis
  - Septicaemia
  - Endotoxaemia
- Metabolic
  - Starvation/ketoacidosis
  - Heat stroke

- Toxic
  - Lead
  - Endotoxaemia
- CNS compression
  - Traumatic (concussion, cranial or spinal fracture)
  - Degenerative (disc prolapse)

KEY HISTORY

- Age at onset
- Duration and progression
- Possible access to lead, occurrence of trauma, or exposure to excessive heat
- Associated clinical signs
  - Gastrointestinal signs
  - Behavioural changes
  - Anorexia
  - Incomplete ingestion of caecotrophs
  - Inadequate grooming
  - Urine scalding as a result of abnormal posturing for micturition

PHYSICAL EXAMINATION

- Distinguish where possible between pure ataxia and other neurologic syndromes such as vestibular disease, paresis, seizures, etc.
- Full physical and neurological examination, particularly to differentiate between primary neurological disease and neurological disease secondary to another (anorexia, infectious, toxic, respiratory) disease process

DECISION-MAKING

- Are clinical signs of sufficient severity/ duration to warrant euthanasia?

- Is the ataxia progressing, decreasing or recurrent?
- Is general supportive therapy indicated?

DIAGNOSTIC APPROACH

- Haematology and biochemistry
- Urine trichrome stained cytology (poorly sensitive but immediate test for *Encephalitozoon cuniculi*)
- *Encephalitozoon cuniculi* serology
- Serum lead evaluation
- Spinal radiography +/– myelography
- CSF analysis (particularly for signs of inflammatory disease)
- CT/MRI

BEHAVIOURAL CHANGES

As with dogs and cats, rabbits can suffer from primary behaviour abnormalities, but also changes in behaviour, especially sudden changes, can be a sign of clinical disease conditions and should be investigated to rule these out before a diagnosis of primary 'behavioural problems' is made. Full discussion of primary behavioural problems is beyond the scope of this text – the reader is referred particularly to www.rabbit.org/behavior/index.html for further information.

The conditions listed below give a rough guide to common medical conditions associated with behavioural changes, but this list is by no means exhaustive.

Common behavioural changes which can be associated with organic disease

- Reluctance to move or to exercise, dullness depression and lethargy
- Circling, reluctance to turn in one direction or inability to turn around
- Inability to recognize owners (with or without nervousness or aggression)
- Alteration in appetite

- Altered urination site, posture, timing
- Tremor, stiffness, apparent ataxia
- Apparent deafness

Medical conditions which can have behaviour changes as a major clinical sign

- Metabolic disease (uraemia, hepatic encephalopathy, ketosis)
- Encephalitozoonosis
- Other CNS lesions
  - Encephalitis
  - Neoplasia
  - Disc prolapse
  - Post-anaesthetic cognitive dysfunction
- Otitis media/interna, *Psoroptes* ear mite infestation
- Toxicity
  - Enterotoxaemia
  - Lead toxicity
  - Carbon monoxide
  - Ototoxic drugs
  - Toxic plants
- Hypoxaemia in advanced respiratory or cardiac disease
- Any painful disease condition

BLEEDING/COAGULOPATHIES

Clotting mechanisms and coagulation disorders have been well studied in rabbits, both as a model for human coagulation disorders and for investigations into the effects of anticoagulant rodenticides.

Although an inherited bleeding disorder similar to von Willebrand disease has been identified in an inbred strain of laboratory rabbits, other inherited or acquired bleeding disorders appear to be rare.

- Rodenticide poisoning – rabbits have a variable and genetically determined resistance to warfarin toxicity
- Viral haemorrhagic disease
- Disseminated intravascular coagulopathy as a consequence of septicaemia or toxaemia

CAECOTROPH ACCUMULATION

Rabbits should produce caecotrophs once or twice daily as part of the 'soft faeces' phase of their digestive cycle. These should be eaten directly from the anus, not from the ground, with the rabbit's head bent down between its legs. Although this caecotrophy behaviour may occasionally be observed by the owner, the caecotrophs themselves should never be seen.

Accumulation of caecotrophs can be divided into conditions leading to relative excess (i.e. more produced than the rabbit chooses to consume) and conditions resulting in physical inability to ingest them. In addition, their nature may be altered, both reducing actual intake, and making them stickier and more difficult to eat whole. The two former situations can co-exist and act synergistically; for example, a rabbit fed to excess with concurrent mild dental pain will be more likely to accumulate caecotrophs than a rabbit with only one factor present. Given the interrelationship between diet and dental and GI health, more than one factor is likely to be involved.

Conditions resulting in excessive production relative to consumption

- Excessive protein levels in the food.
- Excessive carbohydrate/sugar levels in the food.

- Excessive amounts of highly palatable food offered.
- Inadequate fibre intake in the food.
- Change in diurnal routine.
- Stress and unexpected changes to routine may disturb the rabbit sufficiently to momentarily interfere with caecotrophy. An isolated incident is unlikely to be a problem.
- Certain herbs and legumes decrease palatability of caecotrophs. This may be a temporary effect – feeding lettuce to a rabbit unaccustomed to it makes the caecotrophs taste more bitter, but if fed regularly the rabbit will learn to accept the new taste.

Conditions resulting in inability to ingest
Animal factors
- Obesity (+/– large dewlaps or ventral abdominal skin folds)
- Spinal disease (e.g. spondylitis, kyphosis)
- Abdominal pain or large mass
- Dental disease (pain or difficulty prehending the caecotrophs)
- Painful perineal region (e.g. urine scald, dermatitis, myiasis, infected or large skin folds)
  - Contact with wet or dirty floors
  - PU/PD
  - Inability to clean area sufficiently, i.e. vicious cycle develops

DIFFERENTIAL DIAGNOSIS

- Pododermatitis, making it painful for rabbit to change position to reach anus
- Long coat or inadequate grooming (e.g. Angora rabbits)
- Use of 'Elizabethan' type collars
- Neurological disease (e.g. *Encephalitozoon cuniculi*) affecting mobility or balance
- Inadequate exercise
- Too small a hutch or cage to allow the rabbit to reach its anus
- Slippery flooring affecting balance
- Any other condition causing low grade discomfort, lethargy or inability to reach anus (e.g. other musculoskeletal disorders)

Caecotroph factors
- Decreased fibre intake leads to increased stickiness, making them difficult to ingest
- Other enteric disease may alter consistency and composition

These syndromes are rarely fatal in themselves, but may be chronically unpleasant, may indicate a more serious underlying condition, and may predispose to localized dermatitis or myiasis (see Myiasis, p. 49).

Diagnosis and treatment regimes are described under specific chapter headings. Generally an improvement in diet, increased activity (p. 51), and treatment of any underlying pathology (where possible) corrects the problem, although it may take weeks to months to effect a cure.

Treatment of any inflamed skin is advised, to avoid further progression of the disorder, and to reduce the risk of flystrike (see Myiasis, p. 49).

Immediate treatment
- Analgesia, antibiotics, gentle clipping and cleaning of the inflamed skin

Treatment of chronic cases
- If there is an underlying digestive, dental, urogenital or musculoskeletal cause, this should be addressed as detailed in the specific chapters
- Long coated breeds require regular trimming
- Rabbits with incisor dental disorders, or no incisors, may require regular grooming of the perineal area
- Rabbits with skin folds may benefit from corrective surgery

CARDIAC MURMURS AND DYSRHYTHMIAS

With the exception of atherosclerosis (for which the rabbit has been used as a model of human disease), there is relatively little information available regarding cardiac disease in the rabbit. With recent advances in healthcare and husbandry, rabbits can be expected to live longer and often with a greater degree of freedom to exercise than with the traditional hutch bound animal. It is likely that cardiac disease will become a more commonly recognized problem in the rabbit. Much of the following is based on the approach to canine or feline patients with similar presentation.

PRESENTATION

- Clinically healthy but a murmur or dysrhythmia noted during routine examination or during anaesthetic monitoring
- Evidence of congenital cardiac disease
  - Failure to thrive, failure to gain weight
  - Collapse
- Evidence of decompensated cardiac disease
  - Weakness, lethargy
  - Weight loss
  - Dyspnoea

○ Collapse
○ Abdominal distension
• Concurrent disease which is affecting cardiac function

CLASSIFICATION

Murmurs
• Intensity graded I–VI
• Point of maximum intensity and radiation
• Timing and duration, pitch, gallop beats, etc. are usually very difficult to determine because of the normally very rapid heart rate (130–325 beats/minute), especially in small breeds

Dysrhythmias
Unless severe, dysrhythmias are difficult to characterize or even appreciate on auscultation – electrocardiography is usually necessary.

KEY HISTORY

• Age and breed
  ○ Cardiomyopathy seen, especially in giant rabbits
  ○ Some laboratory rabbit breeds are specifically susceptible to atherosclerosis (e.g. Watanebe displays hypercholesterolaemia even on extreme low fat diets)
  ○ Congenital defects such as ventricular septum defects can affect rabbit kits, but rabbit kits with apparently innocent murmurs also occur
• Diet
  ○ Vitamin E deficiency can cause cardiomyopathy
  ○ High fat diets can induce atherosclerosis
  ○ Excessive calcium and vitamin D_3 supplementation may be a cause of aortic mineralization

• Access to potential toxins
  ○ Foxglove (cardiac glycosides)
  ○ Deadly nightshade (atropine; but most rabbits are resistant due to circulating atropinesterase)
  ○ Others
• Previous disease history
  ○ Rabbits surviving *Salmonella*, *Pasteurella* and Tyzzer's disease infections can have cardiomyopathy
  ○ Encephalitozoonosis can be a cause of cardiomyopathy and possibly of dysrhythmia
  ○ Renal disease can result in hypercalcaemia with consequent aortic mineralization
• Anaesthetic history
  ○ Excessive stimulation by adrenaline and α_2-adrenoceptor agonists has been suggested as possible causes of cardiomyopathy

PHYSICAL EXAMINATION

• Where possible, characterization of murmur and rhythm
• Mucosal colour
  ○ Difficult to assess in many breeds
  ○ Iris colour in albino breeds
  ○ Vulva/prepuce
  ○ Pulse-oximetry
• Assessment of peripheral circulation
  ○ Warmth of feet and ear tips
  ○ Capillary refill time
  ○ Pulse quality
  ○ Blood pressure measurement
• Respiratory rate +/– dyspnoea
• Ascites or ventral/peripheral oedema
• Exophthalmos
• Signs of other disease processes

DECISION-MAKING

• Is this an incidental finding; is it congenital?

- Is this secondary to some other disease process (e.g. anaemia, pyrexia, toxaemia, ketosis)?
- Are there clinical signs of cardiac disease?

DIAGNOSTIC APPROACH

- Electrocardiography

- Echocardiography
- Haematology and biochemistry to rule out systemic disease, assess renal function, look for signs of inflammatory disease
- Thoracic radiography, but this will require general anaesthesia which could exacerbate clinical cardiac disease

COLLAPSE/SYNCOPE

'Collapse' is a common presenting syndrome in rabbits. Often it is not a primary symptom, but rather the endstage of one of a wide range of disease processes. A comprehensive investigative process is necessary to attempt to ascertain the primary cause of collapse.

BROAD CATEGORIES OF COLLAPSE

Cardiovascular
- Congestive failure
- Dysrhythmia
- Pericardial disease
- Mediastinal disease (thymoma, abscess)
- Electrocution

Haematological
- Anaemia
  - Common as a secondary product of many other diseases
- Haemorrhage
  - Traumatic
  - Neoplastic
  - Coagulopathy (calicivirus, rodenticides)
- DIC
- Endometrial venous aneurysm

Musculoskeletal
- Fracture
- Pain

Metabolic
- Heat stroke
- Hypovolaemia
- Energy metabolism disturbance
  - Hypoglycaemia
  - Volatile fatty acid balance disturbance
- Hypokalaemia
- Hepatic encephalopathy
- Pregnancy toxaemia
- Dystocia
- Diabetic ketoacidosis

Neurological
- Encephalitozoonosis
- Seizure
- Neurotoxin
  - Organochlorine
  - Heavy metal
  - 'Lettuce poisoning' (lactucarium)
- Muscular dystrophy
  - Deficiency of vitamins E or A

Respiratory
- Airway obstruction
- Pleural disease

Pharmacological
- Sedative or anaesthetic agents

Idiopathic
- 'Floppy bunny syndrome'

KEY HISTORY

- Timing of onset
- Dietary history
- Husbandry
- Use of, or access to potential toxins (pesticides, herbicides, etc.)
- Mental status

Timing of episode
- Single vs. recurrent
- Duration
- Timing (with relation to time of day, activity, feeding/digestive physiology pattern)

During the episode
- Is there loss of consciousness?
- Lethargy/disorientation/ataxia
- Concurrent signs of pain, respiratory difficulty, altered defecation/caecotrophy pattern
- Muscular activity (tonic/clonic)?

After the episode
- Time to full recovery
- Gradual vs. sudden recovery
- Postictal behaviour
- Is there return to normality between episodes?

PHYSICAL EXAMINATION

Full clinical examination in an attempt to determine any underlying disease process is mandatory. Particularly observe mentation, attitudes towards feeding, faecal output, respiratory state and neurological examination.

DECISION-MAKING

- Have any underlying disease processes been identified?
- What further investigations are indicated?
- Which investigations need to be performed before supportive treatment is instituted?
- Which investigations can be performed without the need for chemical restraint?
- What is the likelihood of successful diagnosis or of successful treatment (with or without investigations)?

DIAGNOSTIC APPROACH

- Haematology and biochemistry, including electrolytes
- Survey radiographs of abdomen, thorax and skull
- Oral examination while under sedation or anaesthesia
- Echocardiography
- Encephalitozoal serology
- MRI

CONSTIPATION

True constipation, as seen as a consequence of dietary, mobility, obesity or neurological factors in canine and feline patients, does not occur as a simple entity in the rabbit.

Rabbits presented by the owner as 'constipated' are likely to have either accumulation of uneaten caecotrophs around the vent (anus) (see Caecotroph accumulation, p. 13) or else have stopped producing faecal pellets altogether (see Gastrointestinal stasis, p. 31).

DIFFERENTIAL DIAGNOSIS

COUGHING

The rabbit generally has a poor cough response when compared to other species. The rabbit is an obligate nasal breather (in a normal rabbit the epiglottis is firmly positioned over the caudal edge of the soft palate) and mouth breathing only occurs in cases of severe dyspnoea. This makes it difficult in practice to differentiate between coughing and sneezing.

CAUSES

- Nasopharyngeal
  - Foreign body
  - Abscess
  - Secretions from rhinitis causing irritation to the larynx
- Laryngeal
  - Granuloma formation
  - Neoplasia
- Tracheal
  - Foreign body
  - Granuloma formation
  - Collapse
  - Neoplasia
- Mediastinum
  - Thymoma
  - Abscess
- Airway disease
  - Inhaled irritants
  - Bronchopneumonia
- Gastrointestinal disease
  - Because of the tight oesophageal sphincter, vomiting or true gastric regurgitation is extremely rare in rabbits. Dysphagia caused by dental disease could lead to aspiration of ingested food. Aspiration pneumonia occasionally occurs in cases of oesophageal disease and terminally in mucoid enteropathy syndrome.

KEY HISTORY

- Husbandry and dietary history (including potential exposure to respiratory irritants)
- Duration, speed of onset and progression of cough
- Seasonality?
- Associated clinical signs
  - Dyspnoea
  - Lethargy
  - Sneezing
  - Nasal discharge
- Nature of cough
  - Often difficult to categorise in rabbits, or even to distinguish from sneezing

DECISION-MAKING

- Is the animal coughing or sneezing?
- Is the cough a true respiratory sign (or could it be secondary to other thoracic disease)?
- Is the cough likely to be of the upper or lower respiratory tract in origin?

DIAGNOSTIC APPROACH

- Full clinical examination including dental examination
- Radiography. (This presents problems. Conscious dorsoventral radiography may be possible, and may assist in assessing some differentials, such as unilateral pleural disease, abscessation, thymoma or advanced metastatic neoplasia, but rarely provides a fully diagnostic radiograph. The decision to proceed with general anaesthesia to enable radiography of inflated dorsoventral and lateral views, together with further diagnostic tests, such as endoscopic examinations or bronchoalveolar lavage, must be made

on an individual case basis, and often empirical symptomatic treatment in an attempt to stabilize the case will have to take precedence.)

- Bronchoalveolar lavage
  - Cytology
  - Bacteriology

- Endoscopic examination
  - Nasal cavity, nasopharynx, larynx, trachea, pleural space
  - Includes taking samples for cytology, bacteriology or histopathology

DIARRHOEA

Diarrhoea is a very common presenting sign in younger rabbits, though it is unusual in adults. It is very frequently confused with caecotroph retention around the anus (see Large intestinal disorders, p. 133).

Many cases of apparent diarrhoea in the rabbit are in fact due to insufficient ingestion of the normally produced caecotrophs; the accumulation of soft uneaten caecotrophs around the anus mimics diarrhoea (see caecotroph accumulation, p. 13). The two syndromes can be differentiated as follows.

Caecotroph accumulation ('clagging')

- Caecotrophs are normal and are usually produced only once or twice daily.
- Should be ingested directly from the anus, with the rabbit bending its head down between its hindlegs to do this, but for a variety of reasons may not be ingested and may remain adherent to the perineal area. Soft but not liquid.
- Covered in thin layer of mucus only.
- Interspersed with normal hard dry pellets, which are not ingested.
- Rabbit is usually otherwise well in itself with good appetite.
- On microscopy contain large numbers of bacteria and yeasts.

Diarrhoea

- Rabbit is usually depressed and anorexic
- Produced throughout the day and night
- Not usually any normal (hard) pellets present

- May be associated with blood or excessive mucus
- Microscopy shows long fibre particles
- May be liquid
- May be foul smelling
- As caecotrophy develops between 3 and 6 weeks of age, diarrhoea is more likely under this age
- True diarrhoea, because of the subsequent alterations in fluid and electrolyte balance over the large gut surface area, and disturbance of GI flora and motility, is a rapidly life threatening condition
- Because one of the first effects is a disturbance of GI motility, enteritis and consequent dehydration will sometimes reach a life-threatening stage without any observable loss of diarrhoea from the anus

CAUSES

Diet

- Any factor that leads to a change in caecal pH and bacterial flora
  - Sudden dietary changes
  - Inadequate fibre, particularly a problem with cereal based 'mix' type diets
  - High levels of carbohydrates, especially simple sugars, particularly a problem with cereal based 'mix' type diets
  - High levels of protein, a problem with some 'mix' and 'pelleted' diets
  - Food spoilage or fermentation, e.g. grass clippings

Parasites

With the exception of coccidiosis (which is discussed separately below), GI parasite infestations are an uncommon cause of diarrhoea.

- *Graphidium strigosum* (trichostrongyloid stomach worm)
  - Usually asymptomatic
  - Causes weight loss, anaemia and death in high numbers
- *Passalurus ambiguus* and less commonly *P. nonanulatus* (caecal and colonic pinworm)
  - Even in high numbers non-pathogenic, although may lead to overgrooming of the rectal area
  - May be beneficial to digestion
  - Not susceptible to ivermectin

Coccidiosis

Hepatic coccidiosis

- Caused by *Eimeria stiedai* only
- Some diarrhoea secondary to severe hepatic function alteration, biliary obstruction and ascites development
- More commonly presents as general stunting and in severe cases death from hepatic failure

Intestinal coccidiosis

- Eleven species of very variable pathogenicity and site of infection
- Clinical infection can occur at any age but stunted growth is the most common symptom
  - Most noticeable in young rabbits shortly after weaning
- Diarrhoea, usually mild and intermittent, with or without mucus and/or blood
- Can progress to weight loss, dehydration, intussusception, rectal prolapse and death
- Clinical disease can occur before oocysts are present in the faeces

Diagnosis

- Faecal microscopy
- Coccidia often present as subclinical infestations
- Important to demonstrate extremely high numbers of oocysts in faeces or intestinal contents, or moderate numbers of a recognised pathogenic species (e.g. *E. residua*, *E. magna*) in conjunction with (usually post mortem) localization of lesions
- Gross and histopathological post-mortem examination of intestinal epithelium

Cryptosporidiosis

- *Cryptosporidium parvum* can cause transitory diarrhoea in unweaned rabbits, which is self-limiting but retards growth rate. Potentially zoonotic to immunocompromised humans.

Diagnosis

- Ileal or jejunal smears or histopathology, but may be incidental finding in adults
- ELISA on faeces

Flagellates

- For example, *Giardia duodenalis*, *Monocercomonas cuniculi*, *Retortamonas cuniculi*, *Isotricha*-like spp. and *Entamoeba cuniculi*
- These species are a normal part of the microbial flora of the caecum
- They would not normally be found in 'hard faeces', and so their presence is merely an indication of either insufficient caecotroph intake or of altered gastrointestinal motility
- They are not usually pathogenic in themselves, although there is a reported case of catarrhal enteritis due to *G. duodenalis*

Yeasts

- The presence of yeasts (*Cyniclomyces* [*Disaccharomyces/Saccharomyces*] *guttulatulus*) in caecal contents and faeces is normal, even in very high numbers;

increases in diarrhoea are a consequence of altered caecal control rather than suggestive of a pathological organism
- Although generally somewhat smaller and much more variable in size, it is easy for inexperienced microscopists to mistake yeasts for coccidial oocysts

Neoplasms
Reported GI neoplasms of rabbits include:
- Intestinal leiomyoma
- Intestinal leiomyosarcoma
- Sacculus rotundus papilloma
- Rectal papilloma
- Bile duct adenoma
- Bile duct carcinoma
- Locally and hepatic metastatic uterine adenocarcinoma

Early complete surgical resection of primary tumours carries a good prognosis, although large intestinal surgery is frequently complicated by the delicacy of the tissues, post-surgical adhesions and ileus.

Intussusception
- Usually secondary to diarrhoea rather than a cause of it.

Bacteria
Disturbance in normal caecal bacterial and protozoal flora can occur for the following reasons:
- Increased caecal pH, favouring clostridial growth, due to:
  - High fermentable carbohydrate diet
  - Low fibre diet (decreased volatile fatty acid production, altered colonic motility pattern)
  - High protein diet (breakdown to ammonia).
- Antibiotic administration (particularly orally, and those selectively affecting Gram positives and anaerobes, e.g. clindamycin, lincomycin, erythromycin, tylosin, penicillins, and cephalosporins).

- Stress (reduces gut motility via adrenergic effects on the fusus coli).
- Concurrent poor hygiene.
- Various clostridia occur naturally in the rabbit GIT. *Clostridium spiroforme*, however, produces iota-like toxin and is highly pathogenic to rabbits. The few weeks immediately post weaning is the most likely time for bacterial enteritis to develop as the caecal microflora are stabilising.

Other bacterial infections
Clostridium piliforme (previously Bacillus piliformis)
- Causal organism of Tyzzer's disease
- Watery diarrhoea progressing to depression and death, especially in weanling rabbits
- Overt disease can develop in response to stress factors
- May cause intermittent diarrhoea in chronically affected surviving rabbits
- Uncommon in pet rabbits
- Classically post-mortem examination reveals severe thickening of the intestinal wall

Salmonella typhimurium
- Uncommon
- Can result in diarrhoea, along with septicaemia, pyrexia, depression and death

Escherichia coli
Neonatal (between the ages of 1 and 14 days)
- Enteropathic strains termed 'Rabbit EPEC'. (Also known as RDEC-1: rabbit diarrhoea *E. coli*.)
- Watery diarrhoea
- *E. coli* is not a normal occupant of the GIT at this age, therefore isolation of the organism is significant
- Mortality approaches 100%
- Survivors may have retarded growth

- Treatment:
  - Mild cases early in disease may recover with aggressive supportive care, probiotics and antibiotics (e.g. potentiated sulphonamides)
- Prevention:
  - Good hygiene
  - Reduced stress

Post weaning (4–8 weeks)
- Less common, as gastric pH too acidic to permit colonization of gut with *E. coli*, except shortly after weaning
  - Usually affects kits immediately post weaning as pH changes from 5–6.5 to 1–2
  - Up to 3 weeks of age, the milk oil clot in the stomach from the dam's milk prevents pathogenic bacterial colonization
  - Strains involved similar to above
  - Mortality approaches 50%
  - Faecal culture of *E. coli* in itself is not diagnostic, as *E. coli* overgrowth can occur secondary to other GI problems
  - Dysbiosis is further encouraged by high protein, high carbohydrate, low fibre diets at this age
- Treatment:
  - As for neonatal dysbiosis
    — Correct diet
    — Transfaunation or proprietary probiotics
- Prevention:
  - Good hygiene
  - Minimized stress
  - Later weaning
  - Treatment of concurrent disease, e.g. coccidiosis

Proliferative enteritis/enterocolitis
Lawsonia intracellularis (intracellular campylobacter-like organism)
- Causes enterocolitis with or without Rabbit EPEC.

- Acute diarrhoea in 2–4 month old rabbits.
- Difficult to eliminate due to intracellular nature of organisms. Also, the most effective (oral macrolide) antibiotics are contraindicated in rabbits. Fluroquinolones are most appropriate, given for at least 14 days.

Viral agents
A coronavirus present in normal adult rabbits can cause diarrhoea in 3–10 week old kits. There is high morbidity (approx. 50%), with most affected animals dying after a 24 hour period of lethargy, diarrhoea and abdominal swelling.

Rotavirus infections are common. Infection with rotavirus alone causes only mild, self-limiting soft or fluid faeces for a few days, but in conjunction with bacterial pathogens or opportunists mortality in rabbits aged 30–80 days can reach 80% following severe anorexia, greenish-yellow watery diarrhoea and dehydration.

Calicivirus can cause diarrhoea, but often death occurs before clinical signs are noted.

Miscellaneous bacterial and viral enteric diseases
- Vibriosis, campylobacter, adenoviruses, parvoviruses and herpes-like viruses have been isolated in colony outbreaks
- Infection is unlikely in individual or small group pet rabbits

Mycobacterium paratuberculosis
- Causal organism of paratuberculosis
- Intermittent diarrhoea may be seen
- On histopathology, granulomatous enteritis is noted

Yersinia pseudotuberculosis
- Causal organism of pseudotuberculosis
- Occasionally causes diarrhoea
- Uncommon in pet rabbits

Enteropathy (see also Large intestinal disorders, p. 133)

'Mucoid enteritis' is a term commonly used to describe diarrhoea of a mucoid consistency, or faeces with a mucoid coating, especially just at or after weaning. It is not a single entity.

Mucoid enteropathy (probably the same syndrome as 'rabbit epizootic enterocolitis' (rabbit enzootic mucoid enteropathy) is widely recognized in commercial breeding units and suspected to be viral in origin).

- Usually occurs within 2 weeks of weaning. Can less commonly affect adult animals, especially the mothers of affected litters.
- Dysautonomia, similar to (though distinct from) grass sickness in horses or Key–Gaskell syndrome in cats.
- Destruction of autonomic innervation to the colon results in a functional obstruction, without any overt inflammation (hence 'enteropathy' rather than 'enteritis').
- The colon continues to secrete mucus and becomes severely distended with a clear, jelly-like content, some of which may or may not be passed via the anus.
- The functional obstruction leads to a classical fluid/gas accumulation within the small intestines and stomach similar to that seen with the distal small intestinal foreign body.
- The caecal wall continues to absorb water so that the caecal content becomes dehydrated and often the caecum is palpable as a hard mass on the ventral floor of an otherwise fluid- and gas-filled abdomen.
- The rabbit often develops polyuria/polydipsia, and the stomach can become so distended that food and water pool in the oesophagus and this can lead to an aspiration pneumonia.
- The vast majority, if not all, cases of true 'mucoid enteropathy' rapidly die of the condition.

Chronic inflammatory disease

- 'Cowpat'-like or large amounts of soft, bulky faeces
- May be associated with other inflammatory conditions
- Possibly associated with post ovarohysterectomy adhesions
- Possibly immune mediated
- May respond to salazopyrin or steroid therapy

Toxicities

- Rabbits are unable to vomit, and so one would expect more clinical problems with plant toxicities than in the dog or cat
- However, rabbits can be quite picky about trying a new food, and appear to subsequently avoid plants tasting unpleasant or causing GI disturbance
- They also appear to be resistant to the toxic effects of many plants which are poisonous to other species, including ragwort
- Ingestion of large amounts of a plant to which the individual rabbit is not accustomed is likely to cause diarrhoea or reduced caecotroph ingestion simply because of the change in diet rather than true toxic effects
- See p. 115, for further information on toxic plants

Systemic disease especially primary or secondary liver disease

- Environment: any significant stressors, including diet change, pain, systemic disease, changes of routine, can cause diarrhoea through adrenergic effects on the fusus coli.

KEY HISTORY

- Age and lactation/weaning status (including length of time post weaning)

- Young animals (especially just post weaning)
  - More likely to be bacterial, coccidial or cryptosporidial, or enteropathies
  - May receive clostridial iota-like toxin via mother's milk
  - Generally less likely to have enteric bacterial disease whilst still suckling
- Acute or chronic?
- Is the rabbit still eating normally?
- Is the rabbit craving fibre?
- Is the rabbit losing weight or failing to grow?
- Recent feeding history and any changes
- Any changes to environment, presence of stressors
- Nature of faecal pellets
  - Soft faeces, watery, presence of blood or mucus. Watery diarrhoea, with or without blood or mucus is suggestive of enterotoxaemia
- Signs of systemic disease
- Recent use of antibiotics
  - Enterotoxaemia can develop up to 3 weeks after withdrawal of the antibiotic
- Polyuria/polydipsia is extremely suggestive of mucoid enteropathy

DECISION-MAKING

- Is this true diarrhoea, or simply inadequate caecotroph ingestion ('clagging') (see above)?
- Is this primarily a GI disease or is the diarrhoea a result of dietary change, systemic disease or environmental stress?

- If the rabbit is systemically well, hydrated, and the diarrhoea mild, is it likely to be self-limiting assuming correction of diet and environment?
- Has previous symptomatic treatment been attempted and failed, necessitating further investigation?

DIAGNOSTIC APPROACH

- Faecal microscopy
- In rabbits within 2–3 weeks post weaning or younger, faecal culture
- Dietary trial on hay/grass and water only for up to 1 month, followed by slow reintroduction of one new foodstuff at a time
- Haematology and biochemistry to exclude systemic disease, especially liver disease
- Full clinical examination including abdominal palpation, percussion and auscultation
- 'Hot water bottle' feel to abdomen suggestive of enterotoxaemia or mucoid enteropathy
  - Indicates fluid–gas interface
- Oral/dental examination, under sedation or GA if necessary
- Gross and histopathological examination of intestine (usually at post mortem) in colonies
  - Clinical signs are not usually diagnostic alone, and gross and histopathological examination of gut wall, combined with intestinal content microscopy at specific sites is often necessary to arrive at a definitive diagnosis in mass mortality/morbidity incidents

DYSPHAGIA

- Defined as difficulty or pain in prehending food or swallowing
- A very common presenting symptom in the rabbit
- The vast majority of cases are due to dental pathology
- Other conditions may be responsible

Oropharyngeal dysphagia

- Due to problems prehending food, forming a food bolus and transferring the bolus to the orophaynx
- By far the most common type, and usually due to tooth pathology or secondary tongue lesions
- Usually associated with reduced food intake, weight loss, or altered food preferences

Pharyngeal dysphagia

- Due to problems co-ordinating the passage of food into the oesophagus
- Much less common, and again most likely due to tooth pathology, both directly and indirectly via soft tissue lesions within the mouth, or abscess formation
- Also laryngeal granulomas

Oesophageal dysphagia

- Disorder of oesophageal motility
- May result in regurgitation and aspiration pneumonia
- Very uncommon

CAUSES

Mouth/face

- Stomatitis/glossitis
  - Caustic
  - Immune mediated
  - Renal failure
  - Teeth associated
  - Electrical burns
- Oral tumour
- Retrobulbar mass
  - Does not seem to interfere with mastication as much as similar lesions in cats/dogs
- Otitis externa
  - Painful lesions in the parotid region may cause pain on mastication
- Foreign body, e.g. hay, grass, grass awn
  - Most common in rabbits with dental disease
- Mandibular fracture or luxation
- Facial nerve paralysis
- Teeth, including iatrogenic trauma during dentistry
- Temporomandibular joint and musculature
  - Trauma, myositis, etc. (e.g. trauma to jaw musculature following dental examination)
- Lip swelling, e.g. myxomatosis, treponematosis
- Dysautonomia

Pharyngeal

- Foreign body, e.g. hay, grass, grass awn
- Most common where dental disease present
- Neoplasia
- Tonsillar inflammation or lymphadenopathy
- Pharyngitis
- Facial nerve damage

Laryngeal

- Trauma, e.g. iatrogenic intubation trauma
- Granuloma formation, +/– foreign body
- Neoplasia
- Oedema
  - Insect bites
  - Anaphylaxis
  - Steroid anaesthesia (alphaxalone/alphadolone mixture; Saffan®)

External oesophageal obstruction/retropharyngeal disease

- Cervical neoplasia, lymphadenopathy or abscessation
- Mediastinal tumours or abscessation
  - Thymic
  - Pericardial or cardiac
- Lung tumour or abscessation

Oesophageal disease

- Oesophagitis
- Oesophageal stricture
- Oesophageal foreign body
- Oesophageal diverticulum or rupture

Other disorders (systemic)

- Myasthenia gravis
- Rabies
  - Not seen in the UK
  - Paralytic rabies may be seen in the USA, usually after contact with affected racoons
- Tetanus
  - No recorded cases in practice
  - Has been induced experimentally
- Botulism
  - No recorded cases in practice
  - Has been induced experimentally
- *Encephalitozoon cuniculi*
- Dysautonomia

KEY HISTORY

- Duration and progression
- Any associated clinical signs
  - Retching
  - Coughing (rare) or sneezing
  - Vomiting or regurgitation (very rare)
  - Hypersalivation (common with oral disease)
- Interest in food
- Eating behaviour
  - Any attempts to eat
  - Dropping food
  - Eating on one side of mouth

- Backing away from food
- Change in food preferences
- Difference in ability to eat and drink, and to drink from bowl vs. drinker
- History of trauma, possibility of foreign body ingestion, e.g. long grass
- Nasal discharge, sneezing, etc.
- Accumulation of caecotrophs
- Dermatological disease due to decreased grooming ability

PHYSICAL EXAMINATION

- Conscious oral/dental examination
- Palpation of head and neck
- Thoracic palpation, auscultation and compression
- Neurological examination, especially with regard to head carriage and nystagmus
- Observation of eating, either in hospital or on video

DECISION-MAKING

- If there are dental abnormalities, do I need to anaesthetize this rabbit and complete my dental examination, or has conscious examination been sufficient to arrive at a hopeless prognosis?
- If there is little or no visible dental abnormality, and no other abnormality on conscious examination, in most cases this will necessitate examination under anaesthesia to work up fully.

DIAGNOSTIC APPROACH

Haematology and biochemistry

- Rule out systemic disease, inflammation, infection, tissue trauma
- Lead toxicology
- Electrolytes: calcium elevated with thymoma

Serology
- *Encephalitozoon cuniculi* (unlikely cause of dysphagia, unless as a result of head tilt)

Examination of oral cavity under general anaesthesia
- To include skull radiography, and full oropharyngeal examination as below

Radiography
- As part of full dental examination
- Head, neck and thorax for space occupying masses

Laryngoscopy
- Examination with laryngoscope, otoscope or endoscope

- Include examination of Eustachian tubes, soft palate for foreign body
- Biopsy of any abnormal tissue
- Endoscopic examination of oesophagus

Ultrasonography
- Of neck, retrobulbar space and thorax for space occupying lesions

Fluoroscopy
- Indicated where oesophageal dysphagia suspected

CT scan
- Indicated for more complete imaging of teeth

DYSPNOEA

Dyspnoea:
- In humans, dyspnoea is described as the sensation of breathlessness
- In animals, dyspnoea is assumed where there is increased respiratory effort and distress, i.e. laboured breathing

Hyperpnoea:
- Increased effort without distress

Tachypnoea:
- Increase in the respiratory rate

TYPES OF DYSPNOEA

Physiological dyspnoea
- Breathlessness occurring after exercise
- Similar response is seen in some rabbits due to the stress of physical examination
- Also seen in rabbits with heat stroke

Pulmonary dyspnoea
- Decreased effective lung volume or functional capacity

Cardiac dyspnoea
- Inadequate oxygen delivery from the lungs to the tissues
  - Cardiovascular disease
  - Anaemia

CAUSES

Non-respiratory causes
- Circulatory disease
  - Anaemia
  - Hypertension
  - Congestive heart failure
  - Carbon monoxide poisoning (rabbits housed in garages)
- Abdominal enlargement
  - Abdominal cavity in rabbits is over three times the size of the thoracic cavity
  - Abdominal disease is common
  - Decreases the ability of the diaphragm to ventilate the lungs fully
- Hyperthermia
  - Rabbits are highly susceptible to heat stroke

DIFFERENTIAL DIAGNOSIS

- Metabolic disturbance
  - Acidosis, hepatic lipidosis and ketosis are common sequels to anorexia
- Stress
  - Anxiety, fear, pain

Upper respiratory tract causes

The rabbit is an obligate nasal breather (in a normal rabbit the epiglottis is firmly positioned over the caudal edge of the soft palate, and mouth breathing only occurs in cases of severe dyspnoea). Upper respiratory tract disease therefore has a more profound effect on overall health than in the dog or cat which would initially simply breathe through the mouth.

- Rhinitis
  - Infectious – *Pasteurella*, *Bordetella*, *Staphylococcus*, myxomatosis
  - Chronic – synergism between bacterial infections leads to an atrophic rhinitis syndrome
- Foreign body
  - Particularly pieces of hay entering via nostril
- Abscessation
  - Foreign body
  - External trauma
  - Alteration of apex of the upper premolars
- Granuloma formation
  - Laryngeal granuloma, possibly associated with foreign body
- Neoplasia
- Tracheal disease
  - Foreign body
  - Neoplasia

Lower respiratory tract causes

- Bronchial disease
  - Chronic bronchitis, usually associated also with rhinitis and bronchopneumonia
- Diseases of the lungs
  - Bronchopneumonia
  - Abscessation
  - Neoplasia
  - Contusion

- Inhaled irritants – e.g. ammonia in soiled hutches, petrol, diesel or solvent fumes in garages
- Paraquat toxicity

Thoracic cavity disease

- Pleural space disease
  - Pneumothorax
  - Pyothorax
  - Haemothorax
  - Chylothorax
  - Ruptured diaphragm
- Mediastinal disease
  - Thymoma
  - Lymphosarcoma: often enlarged mediastinal lymph nodes without peripheral lymphadenopathy
  - Abscess
  - Oesophageal rupture
- Thoracic wall trauma

Other causes

- Musculoskeletal damage
- Pain

KEY HISTORY

- Husbandry and diet
- Duration and speed of onset of clinical signs
- Other associated signs
  - Oculonasal discharge
  - Cough/sneeze
  - Ptyalism
  - Anorexia
- Potential exposure to toxins or irritants
- Similar signs in contact animals

PHYSICAL EXAMINATION

- Observation of respiratory pattern in relaxed animal
  - Within carrier or loose on consulting room floor
- Mucous membrane colour
  - Difficult to assess
  - Iris colour in pink-eyed breeds

- Inspection and palpation of nostrils, facial anatomy, trachea and larynx
- Thoracic auscultation, percussion and compression
- Full clinical examination for potential non-respiratory disease, including thorough dental examination

DECISION-MAKING

- Is the general condition stable?
  - If not, consider placing in a cool oxygen tent and providing appropriate emergency treatments, such as fluid therapy, analgesia.
- Respiratory versus non-respiratory?
  - If non-respiratory causes are suspected, the diagnostic approach may differ from that below.
- If respiratory, upper/lower/both?
- Is the animal's condition stable enough to allow for diagnostic tests?

DIAGNOSTIC APPROACH

- Thoracic radiography. (This presents problems. Conscious dorsoventral radiography may be possible, and may assist in assessing some differentials, such as unilateral pleural disease, abscessation, thymoma or advanced metastatic neoplasia, but rarely provides a fully diagnostic radiograph. The decision to proceed with general anaesthesia to enable inflated dorsoventral and lateral views, together with further diagnostic tests such as endoscopic examinations or bronchoalveolar lavage must be made on an individual case basis; often empirical symptomatic treatment in an attempt to stabilize the case will have to take precedence.)
- Thoracocentesis
  - Diagnostic
  - Therapeutic
- Bronchoalveolar lavage
  - Cytology
  - Bacteriology
- Endoscopic examinations
  - Nasal cavity
  - Nasopharynx
  - Larynx
  - Trachea
  - Bronchi
  - Pleural space
  - With or without sampling for cytology, bacteriology or histopathology
- Cardiac ultrasound
- Haematology and biochemistry

DYSURIA

Dysuria:
- Painful or difficult urination

Pollakiuria:
- Passing frequent small amounts of urine

Stranguria:
- Straining or hesitancy to pass urine

Care must be taken to distinguish dysuria from simple perineal wetting due to immobility, inability to groom or localized (perineal fold) dermatitis. Rabbits can pass frequent small amounts of urine for behavioural reasons also, and this must be differentiated from physiological pollakiuria.

Absence of urination can be due to obstruction, or true oliguria in cases of renal failure.

CAUSES

Inflammatory

- Retention of urine and pain during micturation due to perineal fold dermatitis
- Infectious
  - Bacterial, e.g. *Treponema paraluiscuniculi*
  - Microsporidian, e.g. *Encephalitozoon cuniculi, Toxoplasma gondii*

Neurological

- Spinal trauma
- *Encephalitozoon cuniculi* hindlimb and urinary tract neurological deficits

Musculoskeletal

- Spinal pain, e.g. spondylosis
- Other hindlimb pain or stiffness
- Renal calculi causing paresis due to sub-lumbar pain
- Neuromuscular disease causing skeletal muscle necrosis if exercise severely restricted

Obstructive

- Trauma
- Urolithiasis
- Urinary sludge syndrome
- Upper motor neurone disease
- Urethral muscle spasm/reflex dyssynergia
- Iatrogenic following catheterization, surgery, etc.
- Compression from uterus or local soft tissue mass
  - Hydrometra, pyometra, uterine torsion, dystocia

Anatomic

- Congenital abnormalities
- Acquired abnormalities
  - Urethral stricture
  - Phimosis
  - Bladder evertion
    — Presents as apparent straining to urinate, easily differentiated on clinical examination
  - Neoplastic

KEY HISTORY

- Age, sex, neutered or entire
- Diet and supplementation
- Method of drinking
- Previous history of dysuria
- Is the rabbit passing urine at all?
- If the rabbit is passing urine, is it aware of doing so?

- Other clinical signs (urinary)
  - Pollakiuria
  - Haematuria
  - Loss of litter training
  - Perineal soiling
  - Incontinence
  - Pain associated with urine passage
- Clinical signs of any other disease process
- Duration and progression of clinical signs
- History or evidence of trauma

PHYSICAL EXAMINATION

- Full clinical examination
  - Especially evaluating body condition (obesity, cachexia)
  - For diseases that might cause immobility or decreased grooming
- Abdominal palpation, auscultation and percussion
- How full is the bladder?
  - *Care:* rabbits' bladders are thin walled, can distend enormously and may rupture if handled
- Can urine be expressed?
  - Rabbits normally void urine with light pressure on the bladder
- Examination of external genitalia and urethral opening
- Is there evidence of passive urine overflow or incontinence, e.g. urine staining/scalding?
- General neurological examination
  - Observation of the rabbit moving around on the floor to assess mobility and hindlimb function
- Observation of the rabbit urinating, if possible

DECISION-MAKING

- Is the rabbit obstructed?
- Is emergency bladder decompression indicated?

- Is the bladder intact?
- Is some other process involved, e.g. straining due to vaginal prolapse, faecal tenesmus?

DIAGNOSTIC APPROACH (FOLLOWING DECOMPRESSION IF OBSTRUCTED)

Urinalysis
(Important to allow for method of obtaining sample, especially with culture and sensitivity.)

- Gross appearance
- Biochemistry
- Sediment examination
- Cellular or cast material is usually found at the interface between crystalline sediment and clear supernatant after centrifugation or settlement
- Bacterial culture and sensitivity
- Examination for *Encephalitozoon cuniculi*
  - Trichrome stained sediment cytology

Haematology and biochemistry
- Determination of systemic illness, e.g. renal
- Include total and ionized calcium

Ease of passage of urinary catheter
- Is there a palpable obstruction?

Diagnostic imaging
- Radiography of entire urinary tract on DV and lateral views
- Plain radiographs taking care to avoid disturbance of bladder 'sand'
  - Consider a horizontal beam standing lateral in cases with presumed sludging syndrome to differentiate settled sludge from suspended crystals
- Negative contrast cystography
- Double contrast cystography
- Urethrogram
- Intravenous excretory urograph
- Ultrasound examination of abdomen, including bladder, ureters, kidneys, uterus
- Perurethral uroendoscopy (in the female)
  - Evaluation of urethra and bladder
  - Visualization of ureteral openings
  - Identification and removal of small calculi

Exploratory laparotomy and examination of ureters, bladder, uterus
- Cystotomy, bladder wall examination and biopsy, removal of any calculi for examination
- Biopsy of any abnormal tissue causing extraluminal obstruction

Urolith or calculus examination
- Entire calculus, not just surface

Serology
- *Treponema paraluis-cuniculi*
- *Encephalitozoon cuniculi*
- *Toxoplasma gondii* (much less common)

GASTROINTESTINAL STASIS

Lack of faecal output, either absolute, or by reduction in the size or number of pellets, is a common presenting sign in the rabbit. It tends to go hand in hand with inappetance.

Gut stasis
- Increased gut transit time
- Faeces may be smaller, harder, drier and present in reduced quantities or not at all, corresponding to constipation and obstipation, respectively, in the cat and dog

- There may be passage of liquid or mucus in some cases
- Very common

Megacolon
- Cases of neurological impairment have been recorded, but altered colonic motility with caecal distension is more common than distension of the colon itself
- There may be an increased incidence of true megacolon in white rabbits with dark coloured eyes and dark skin spots

Tenesmus
- Straining to pass faeces
- Uncommon

Dyschezia
- Pain and difficulty when passing or attempting to pass faeces
- Uncommon

CAUSES

Diet (see also Nutrition, p. 105)
Rabbits are an herbivorous prey species. They need to maximize their feeding time in the wild, without increasing their exposure to predators. They have a small body size, and their natural diet is low in energy, fat, protein and digestible carbohydrate, and high in indigestible fibre. They have evolved to deal with these problems by having a fast gut transit time.

The fusus coli, a muscular band of well innervated tissue with a thickened mucosa, lying at the end of the proximal colon, acts as the pacemaker to the colon, which has two distinct phases of motility.
- In the first it channels large particles of indigestible fibre directly to the anus where they are voided in the form of typical rabbit faecal pellets, whilst separating out and retaining small particles and fluid which are passed to the caecum.

- In the second, the end-products of caecal microbial fermentation, the caecotrophs, are produced, which are eaten directly from the anus.
- These pellets pass back through the gut and are digested.
- This complex pattern of gut motility is driven by the presence of high levels of dietary fibre. If those are removed, the system has a tendency to grind to a standstill.

This is the most important concept in understanding gut motility disorders in the rabbit: they are designed to eat grass.

Specific dietary parameters involved in gut stasis are as follows:
- Inappropriately low levels of indigestible fibre (too little to stimulate proper gut motility as above)
- Insufficient long particles of indigestible fibre (too little to stimulate proper gut motility, as above)
- High levels of carbohydrates (especially simple sugars) affecting caecal pH and therefore microbial fermentation
- High levels of protein affecting caecal pH and therefore microbial fermentation
- Ingestion of indigestible particulate matter, especially clay based materials
  - Clay based litter tray substrate
  - Montmorillonite based 'diarrhoea' treatments

Foreign body impaction
There is an historical idea that gut stasis is the result of 'furballs' or 'woolblock'; this is also known as 'trichobezoar' and was thought to occur due to the presence of fur in the stomachs of rabbits with gut stasis. However, the fur is a result of the gut stasis, not the cause. The normal rabbit stomach always contains food, and there is often fur present. Dehydration of this matrix of fur and food leads to the classic appearance of a furball on radiography and at post mortem.

Mats of moulted fur as well as other foreign bodies may, however, occlude the gut. This is covered under acute Obstructive ileus (p. 127).

Foreign bodies commonly include:
- Pieces of carpet
- Clay based cat litter
- Corn cob cat litter
- Discrete mats of fur moulted from rabbit or cagemates. These are especially common in rabbits with dental disease. Fur can build up in solid mats, especially on the feet
- Locust bean pods (less commonly present in foods now but can still occur)
- Corn pips
- Dried peas

(Note that unmatted fur is a normal finding in the rabbit stomach, and if present in large amounts is usually a symptom of gastric stasis rather than a cause.)

Common impaction sites include:
- Pylorus
- Pyloroduodenal angle
- Sacculus rotundus

Environment

It takes very little to stress a rabbit, and catecholamine release, especially in the obese rabbit, acts to decrease gut motility. Any cause of stress can affect rabbits in this way:
- Any source of pain
- Predators and other animals
  - Domestic – cats, dogs, ferrets
  - Wild – foxes, mink, polecats, rodents
- Dominance issues: bullying by another rabbit, or hierarchical disputes
- Sudden diet changes
- Transportation
- Weather or temperature changes
- Loss of companion
- Unavailability of water or food
- Loud noises
  - Fireworks, thunderstorms, gunshots
- Change in routine, e.g. sudden daylength changes
- Trauma

In addition, some environmental factors can specifically hinder the act of defecation:
- Inappropriate litter tray substrate
- Unpleasant weather if litter area is outside
- Pain making it difficult to get to the litter area or to defecate
  - Musculoskeletal pain, e.g. arthritis
  - Foot pain, e.g. plantar pododermatitis
  - Visceral pain, e.g. GI bloating
  - Perineal pain, e.g. urine scalding +/– flystrike
  - Urological pain, e.g. urolithiasis

Neuromuscular disease affecting colonic function
- Spinal or peripheral neuropathy
- Dysautonomia (mucoid enteropathy)

Intraluminal obstruction
- Colonic/rectal neoplasia (rare cause of obstruction)
- Polyps (not uncommonly found, but rare cause of constipation)
- Foreign body (sites of impaction described later)
- Stricture, intussusception, torsion

Extraluminal obstruction
- Narrowed pelvic canal
- Cystic calculi, ano-rectal/perineal mass, e.g. abscess, neoplasia, parasitic cyst
- Perineal hernia

Drugs
- Opioids. Although in theory therapeutic doses of opioid analgesics could slow gut motility, in practice this is extremely unlikely, and generally their analgesic effects help to restore gut motility
- Loperamide (avoid its use in rabbits altogether)

Toxicity
- Lead poisoning causes slow gut motility and unevacuated faeces

DIFFERENTIAL DIAGNOSIS

Dysautonomia (mucoid enteropathy; rabbit epizootic enterocolitis)

- Similar to grass sickness in horses
- Other autonomic signs, e.g. mydriasis, reduced tear production and salivation may be seen
- Diagnosed at histopathology

Other problems

- Inflammation of the gut or associated structures, with or without pain (e.g. gastroenteritis, peritonitis)
- Any severe systemic disease
- Obesity
- Behavioural, e.g. dominant rabbit or predator present in litter area
- Severe electrolyte disturbances may result in altered GI motility
- Dehydration

KEY HISTORY

It is important to differentiate between non-obstructive ileus, described here, and obstructive ileus, which is a more acute condition requiring surgical intervention in conjunction with high levels of medical and nursing support.

Non-obstructive ileus

- A slow, insidious onset
- A gradual decrease in the size of faecal pellets and the frequency of their production
- There may be a craving for high fibre items, not necessarily digestible ones, such as wood, paper, wallpaper, cardboard
- Normal hydration to moderate dehydration
- A normal demeanour at first, becoming gradually depressed and developing abdominal pain later
- Radiographic changes

   - Impacted material in the stomach and caecum
   - There may be a 'halo' of gas around the impacted material
   - Gaseous distension develops as stasis continues, with fluid contents present in the gut in the latter stages

Obstructive ileus

- Sudden onset (over less than 48 hours)
- Rabbits may be found acutely dead with this condition
- A sudden cessation in faecal pellet production
- Moderate to severe depression
- Marked to severe abdominal pain and guarding, with a hunched posture and reluctance to move
- Palpable extreme distension of the stomach
- Shock and severe dehydration
- Radiographic changes
   - Fluid and gas proximal to the site of the obstruction
   - Bubbles of gas rather than a 'halo' in the stomach

DIAGNOSTIC APPROACH

Take a full history, including detailed assessment of diet and environment:
- Food eaten, dietary or appetite changes, possible foreign bodies consumed
- Environment, companion animals, trauma, stress, changes to normal routine, etc.
- Duration
- Presence of tenesmus, dyschezia or haematochezia
- Any possibility of confusion with urinary tenesmus?

Conduct a full clinical examination, including:
- Urinary tract to remove urinary tenesmus as a differential

- Dental examination (under sedation or general anaesthesia as necessary)
- Abdominal palpation, percussion and auscultation
- Examination for any sources of pain or discomfort
- Observation of locomotion
- Examination of any faeces or other material produced

Radiography of:
- Head
- Abdomen

- Spine/pelvis
- Any site of musculoskeletal discomfort

Consider further imaging:
- CT scan of head
- MRI/myelography of spine

Laboratory diagnostics:
- Urinalysis to assist in clarification of urinary tenesmus as a differential
- *Encephalitozoon cuniculi* serology
- Evaluation or cytology of any faecal output

HAEMATOCHEZIA AND MELAENA

Haematochezia and melaena are uncommon presenting signs in rabbits, and can be categorized into visible bleeding, or levels of occult blood only detectable on laboratory analysis.
- Haematochezia: presence of fresh, red blood in faeces, usually from the large intestine
- Melaena: black, tarry faeces resulting from blood digested in the small intestine
  - More difficult to distinguish from normal faeces than in the dog or cat
  - Only likely to be seen in association with diarrhoea or mucoid faeces

HAEMATOCHEZIA

- Neoplasia or polyps, e.g. rectal papillomata
- Rectal/anal trauma
- Colitis
- Typhlitis
- Bleeding disorder (especially terminal rabbit calicivirus infection)

MELAENA

Difficult to identify as normal rabbit faeces are very dark in colour, and caecotrophs

can be dark in colour and tarry in consistency. Bleeding into the gut (e.g. due to ulceration or neoplasia) can be detected by laboratory analysis for faecal occult blood. However, blood will be utilized as a substrate by caecal microbial populations, and it is unlikely that small amounts of blood produced proximally to the caecum will lead to a positive result.
- Infectious disease, e.g. VHD
- Bleeding disorder
- Iatrogenic, e.g. NSAIDs, glucocorticoids
- DIC
- Deficiency of niacin or vitamin K
  - Requires severely deficient diets and absence of caecotrophy
  - Not likely in a pet rabbit situation.
- False positives due to, e.g. horseradish or radish in diet

KEY HISTORY

- Age
- Sex, entire or neutered
- Weaning status
- Access to toxins, especially anticoagulants
- Access to drugs, especially NSAIDs and glucocorticoids
- VHD vaccination status and history of exposure to infected rabbits

- Any recent environmental stress
- Appetite
- Weight loss
- Evidence or history of trauma, including self trauma
- Volume of blood produced
- Is the blood around the pellet or mixed through it?
- Is there concurrent diarrhoea or mucoid faeces?
- Other clinical signs of blood loss
- Is the rabbit systemically ill?
- Is the rabbit showing any signs of lameness?

PHYSICAL EXAMINATION

- Mucosal colour and CRT
- Petechiation or ecchymosis
- Full oral/dental examination
- Auscultation of lung fields
- Abdominal palpation, auscultation and percussion
- Examination of anus
- Palpation and manipulation of joints for swelling or pain

DECISION-MAKING

- Is any blood being lost? Is this a false positive for occult blood in the faeces?
- Has a significant amount of blood been lost?
- Is there evidence of a generalized bleeding disorder?
- Where is the blood originating from?
- Are the blood losses ongoing?

DIFFERENTIAL DIAGNOSIS OF DARK FAECES

- Normal appearance (see above)
- Dietary pigments

- Drugs, e.g. activated charcoal

DIAGNOSTIC APPROACH

Haematochezia
- Faecal (gross and microscopic) examination
- Haematology
  - Be aware that anaemia is a common finding in ill rabbits and does not necessarily confirm ongoing blood loss
- Assessment for bleeding disorders
- Cytology and/or biopsy of any abnormal rectal tissue
- Abdominal radiography
- Proctoscopy and biopsy as necessary
  - *Beware*: the thin-walled nature of the rabbit rectum and colon make proctoscopy a high-risk procedure; consider exploratory laparotomy to examine colon before proceeding

Melaena
- Faecal (gross and microscopic) examination
- Haematology
  - Be aware that anaemia is a common finding in ill rabbits and does not necessarily confirm ongoing blood loss
- Assessment for bleeding disorders
  - History of access to toxins
  - Bruising, subcutaneous bleeding, petechiation or ecchymosis
  - Laboratory assessment of clotting factors
- Biochemistry
  - Causes of ulceration, e.g. uraemia
- Thoracic radiology and ultrasonography
- Abdominal radiography (plain and contrast)
- Exploratory laparotomy and biopsy

HAEMATURIA

Haematuria is a common presenting sign in the rabbit. However, it is first necessary to differentiate genuine haematuria from the presence of red pigmentation in the urine. This can be achieved by the use of dipstick tests (e.g. Multistix, Bayer) to determine the presence of blood or haemoglobin. Alternatively, samples can be centrifuged and examined for the presence of red blood cells. The former test can also be carried out on samples of urine-contaminated bedding placed in a universal container with water. In addition, some urinary pigments fluoresce on exposure to UV light.

Red urine not containing blood

- Urine may be coloured red due to ingested plant material containing porphyrins, such as:
  o Beetroot
  o Cabbage
  o Broccoli
  o Dandelions
  o Pine needles
  o Carrots
  o Acorns
  o Alfalfa
  o *Leucaena*
  o Pigments in pellet or biscuit dietary components
- Urine coloration can occur in one or more of a group of rabbits all fed the same food
- Porphyrin excretion may increase with stress or other concurrent disease
- Dehydration may concentrate the urine, leading to more evident coloration
- Urine coloration may be due to urobilinuria, which appears grossly similar, and can be differentiated on dipstick examination
- Porphyria has been reported in one NZW rabbit. This caused no clinical signs, but at post mortem there was a pink tinge to the teeth, and ultraviolet fluorescence of teeth and bones

- Some antibiotics may cause urine discoloration
- False positives on dipsticks
  o Ascorbic acid
  o Formalin
  o Blood from catheterization or cystocentesis trauma

True haematuria

Site of bleeding: urinary tract
Renal
- Acute pyelonephritis (associated with pyuria)
- Glomerulopathy (may be associated with presence of protein; however, proteins may be seen in the urine of healthy rabbits)
- Neoplasia
- Nephrolithiasis
- Septicaemia
- Terminal VHD
- Infarction
- Trauma
- Herbicide or anticoagulant rodenticide toxicity

Lower urinary tract
- Trauma (falls are the most common cause)
- Calculi
- Urinary tract infection
- Neoplasia
- Polyps in bladder or vagina

Site of bleeding: genital tract
- Neoplasia
- Trauma
- Infection
  o Bacterial
  o *Treponema paraluis-cuniculi*
- Uterine bleeding
  o Hyperplasia
  o Aneurysm
  o Polyp
  o Dystocia

- ○ Prolapse
- ○ Abortion or stillbirth
- ○ Abscess/pyometra
- Vaginal bleeding from prolapse or polyp

Haematuria secondary to systemic disease

- Bleeding disorder
  - ○ e.g. VHD, DIC
  - ○ Other coagulopathy or anticoagulant toxicity
  - ○ Septicaemia
- Hyperthermia
- Exercise/exertional myopathy

KEY HISTORY

- Is this true haematuria?
- Sex
- Neutered or not?
- Previously mated?
- Does the rabbit appear to be in oestrus or not?
- Pregnant (current or recent) or not?
- Is there previous history of haematuria?
- At what stage in urination does the blood appear?
- Is there bleeding every time the rabbit urinates?
- Is there bleeding from the external genitalia not associated with urination?
- Is there any haemorrhage from other sites?
- Are there any other urinary or genital tract signs, e.g. dysuria, perineal scalding?
- Is there concurrent mastitis?
- History, evidence or suspicion of trauma (e.g. two unrelated entire bucks recently introduced together)
- Any similar signs in in-contact rabbits?

PHYSICAL EXAMINATION

- Mucosal colour and CRT
- Petechiation or ecchymosis of skin or mucous membranes

- Palpation, auscultation and percussion of the abdomen
  - ○ Particularly palpation of bladder and uterus
- Examination of external genitalia
- Examination of mammary glands (female)

DECISION-MAKING

- Is this definitely blood and not urinary pigmentation?
- Has a significant amount of blood been lost?
- Is there any evidence of a bleeding disorder?
  - ○ Bleeding, bruising or petechiation elsewhere in the body
- Where is the blood coming from: urinary tract or genital tract?
- Is there any evidence of external genitalia trauma or disease?

DIAGNOSTIC APPROACH

- Urinalysis, including comparison of free catch or collected urine vs. cystocentesis to localize bleeding to urinary tract (especially in entire female)
  - ○ Biochemistry
  - ○ Crystal analysis (but normally high calcium salt crystalluria)
  - ○ Sediment analysis (cytology)
    - — Red cell casts suggest renal disease
    - — White cell casts and bacteria
    - — Neoplastic epithelial cells
  - ○ Bacterial culture and sensitivity
  - ○ *Encephalitozoon cuniculi* microscopy
- Assessment for bleeding disorders
- Examination of external genitalia (including biopsy or skin scrape for *Treponema paraluis-cuniculi*)
- Ultrasound examination of bladder, kidneys and uterus

- Ultrasonography of the bladder after gently shaking the rabbit may reveal calculi that have been displaced and float for a while before settling
- Radiography of bladder, kidneys and uterus
  - Plain radiography
  - Negative contrast cystography
  - Double contrast cystography
  - Retrograde urethrography
  - Intravenous excretory urography
- Haematology and biochemistry
- Serology (*Treponema paraluis-cuniculi*, *Encephalitozoon cuniculi*)
- Endoscopic examination of vagina, urethra, bladder (females only)
- Exploratory laparotomy
  - Cystotomy, biopsy, bladder lavage and examination for calculi
  - Examine uterus, biopsy or ovario-hysterectomy and histopathology

HAEMOPTYSIS

Haemoptysis is coughing and expectorating blood. This is very uncommon in rabbits. Because rabbits are obligate nasal breathers, haemoptysis usually presents as bleeding from the nostril and is difficult to differentiate from true epistaxis. Rabbits have a poor cough reflex and any true coughing (as opposed to sneezing or snorting) carries a poor prognosis. In the vast majority of cases, apparent haemoptysis is likely to be blood in saliva, from an intra-oral lesion.

Haematemesis refers to the vomiting of blood. True vomiting in the rabbit has only very rarely been even anecdotally reported, and there are no reports of haematemesis. Regurgitation of blood from an oesophageal lesion might be possible.

SOURCE OF BLOOD

- Nasopharynx
- Oral cavity
- Oesophagus
- Stomach (rare/non-existent, see above)
- Respiratory tract

CAUSES

- Laryngeal granuloma (possibly foreign body related)
- Bleeding disorder
- Trauma
- Ulceration of oesophagus or stomach
- Foreign body
- Dental disease with laceration of mucosa or discharging abscess
- Neoplasia
- Iatrogenic
- Viral (VHD)

KEY HISTORY

- Age
- Duration and progression of clinical signs
- Clinical signs in contact animals
- Access to anticoagulants, caustic chemicals or NSAIDs
- Appetite
- Weight loss
- Evidence of or history of trauma
- Volume of blood produced
- Nature of blood
  - Fresh, changed
  - Arterial, venous, clotted
  - Presence of pus, mucus, etc. This is often not possible to assess as the material is rarely produced in its original form, as would be the case in canine or feline cases, but has usually been retained within the oral cavity or nasopharynx for some time before being expelled

- Other clinical signs related to a respiratory tract, GIT or coagulopathy disorder
- Any other clinical signs

PHYSICAL EXAMINATION

- Mucosal colour and capillary refill time
- Petechiation or ecchymosis
- Oral and dental examination, under sedation or GA as necessary
- Auscultation of thorax

DECISION-MAKING

- Where is the blood coming from?
- Is there a bleeding disorder?
- Has a significant amount of blood been lost?
- Are blood losses ongoing?

DIAGNOSTIC APPROACH

- Full haematology
- Laboratory assessment of clotting factors
- Biochemistry to explore causes of any ulceration
- Serology or PCR techniques
  - VHD, though unusual for clinical case to survive until results available
- Full oropharyngeal examination under sedation/GA as necessary
- Thoracic radiology
- Rhinoscopy, tracheoscopy (be aware of the normal highly vascular nature of the rabbit trachea) and bronchoscopy, endoscopic examination of the pharynx and oesophagus
- Biopsy of abnormal tissue, and impression cytology or histopathological examination
- Bronchoalveolar lavage/transtracheal lavage

HEAD TILT

'Head tilt' is probably the most commonly presenting neurological symptom seen in rabbits. Severity can vary from slight dropping of one side of the face to rotations of 180° or more. Whilst rabbits can sometimes seem otherwise totally unaffected, it can be associated with extreme balance deficits and can be very distressing for owner and rabbit.

Head tilt is often referred to as torticollis, but this term specifically refers to a contracture of cervical musculature, whereas the majority of head tilt cases are due to disturbances of balance.

CAUSES

Peripheral vestibular disease
Otitis interna or media
- Simple otitis media is *not* usually associated with a full head tilt unless it has progressed to involve the inner ear also

  - May show facial paralysis or Horner's syndrome – ear, eyelid and lip drooping may simulate head tilt appearance
  - May hold head tilted as a consequence of middle/outer ear pain
  - Deafness extremely difficult to assess in rabbits
- Extension of otitis externa
  - Bacterial
  - Parasitic (*Psoroptes cuniculi*)
- Ascending upper respiratory tract infection
  - Bacterial
  - Mycoplasmal
- Foreign body migration through tympanum or iatrogenic aural lesion

Central vestibular disease
Bacterial respiratory tract pathogens
- *Pasteurella*, *Bordetella* and *Staphylococcus*
- (Extension of otitis interna through to brain)

Bacterial encephalitis
- *Listeria monocytogenes*

Parasitic
- *Baylisascaris procyonis* (USA)
- Other ascarids

Protozoal
- Granulomatous meningoencephalitis
- *Encephalitozoon cuniculi* (and rarely *Toxoplasma gondii*)

Viral (herpes virus encephalitis)
- *Herpes simplex 1* has been reported as a cause of circling and spinning in rabbits
- It may be transmitted from humans to rabbits

Non-cranial causes
- Hepatic disease

Less common causes
- Neoplasia
- Cerebrovascular emboli
- Head/neck trauma, especially predation
- Cerebral mycoses
- Toxicosis (lead and some plant toxins)

KEY HISTORY

- Age
- Breed
- Indoor or outdoor rabbit
- Lone rabbit or not?
- History of any neurological disease in in-contact rabbits or parents
- Recent history or evidence of trauma
- Possibility of exposure to lead
- Possibility of exposure to plant toxins, e.g. *Asclepias eriocarpa* (woolly pod milkweed) (USA only)
- History of previous head tilt
- History of respiratory tract disease
- History of aural disease
- Any signs of other clinical disease, especially other neuromuscular disease

- Duration, degree and progression of head tilt
- Dysuria, incontinence
- Contact with human with active herpesviral lesion

PHYSICAL EXAMINATION

- Degree of head tilt
- Does the rabbit also fall over?
- Side to which head tilts
- Presence of nystagmus
  - Vertical or horizontal
  - Continuous, spontaneous or positionally triggered
  - Direction of slow phase
- Other neuromuscular signs, especially hindlimb paresis/paralysis
- Examination for urine soaking or scalding
- Signs of aural disease
- Signs of respiratory disease
- Full opthalmological examination
- Examination of soft tissues of neck and head for puncture wounds

DECISION-MAKING

- Is the rabbit able to eat and drink unaided?
- Is there an increased need for grooming and ectoparasite control?
- Can this be diagnosed as *Encephalitozoon cuniculi*, otitis media/interna or other causes?
- Is the rabbit systemically unwell?

DIAGNOSTIC APPROACH

Correlation with clinical signs
- Head theoretically down on side of lesion
- Vertical nystagmus and positionally triggered nystagmus are more typical of central vestibular disease

- Horizontal nystagmus and spontaneously occurring nystagmus are more typical of peripheral vestibular disease
- Slow phase typically towards the side of the lesion

Clinical pathology

- Full haematology including cell morphology
- Biochemistry, especially renal and hepatic parameters
- Serology for *Encephalitozoon cuniculi*
  - IFAT
  - Rising titres and differentiated IgG and IgM more useful than single test
  - Initially IgG and IgM are elevated
  - IgG decreases and IgM increases during course of an infection
- Lead toxicology

- Microbiological culture of any abscess capsule

Imaging

- Plain radiographs of skull to examine tympanic bullae
  - Lateral, DV and both oblique views. Open mouth skyline view is not usually necessary in rabbits because the tympanic bullae show up well on lateral and DV views
- Survey radiographs for presence of lead
  - Absence of metallic particles does not rule out lead toxicity
- Otoscopic endoscopy to examine tympanic membrane
- CT of skull
- MRI of skull

INFERTILITY – GENERAL

Infertility is an uncommon presenting sign in companion animal practice. Where the emphasis is on prevention of breeding, causes of infertility are likely to be overlooked, or masked by imposed population control. It is economically more notable in breeding systems, and may be an early warning of more serious disease.

REPRODUCTIVE PHYSIOLOGY

- No true 'oestrus cycle'; receptive periods of 7–10 days followed by 1–2 day period of inactivity as new follicles develop
- Induced ovulators
- Reproductive activity in females is suppressed by short day length and low temperatures

EITHER SEX

- Inadequate diet (protein, hypovitaminosis A, D, E, hypervitaminosis A)
- Nitrate contamination of water or food supply
- Obesity (lack of fertility and embryonic resorption)
- Insufficient exercise
- Immaturity
  - 16–24 weeks
  - Smaller breeds mature earliest, as early as 8 weeks with some bucks
- Old age
  - Over 2–3 years in does
  - 5–6 years in bucks
- Trauma/inflammation of external genitalia, e.g. *Treponema paraluis-cuniculi*
- Concurrent disease (systemic or genital)
- Short daylength, low temperature, i.e. winter conditions
- Heat stress
- Environmental disturbance

- Failure of coitus due to musculoskeletal problems
  - Spondylosis/osteoarthritis, etc.
  - Pododermatitis
  - Paresis
- Pair related
  - Incorrect sexing
  - Incompatibility between individuals
  - Aggression between individuals

INFERTILITY – FEMALE

As for General Infertility above, and also:
- Recent parturition
  - Lactating does show delayed implantation
- Prior reproductive tract surgery
  - Including OVH!
- Late first breeding
  - Over 2 years
- Lack of oestrus behaviour if kept as single doe
- Ovarian hypoplasia or aplasia
- Intersex or hypogonadia
- Age-related uterine changes
  - Endometrial hyperplasia
  - Neoplasia
  - Cystic changes
  - Polyps
- False pregnancy
  - Does are not receptive to the buck during false pregnancy
- Ectopic/extrauterine pregnancy
- Systemic or genital tract disease
  - Endometritis (e.g. *Pasteurella multocida*, *Staphylococcus aureus*)
  - *Listeria* infection
  - *Treponema* infection
  - Pyometra (*Pasteurella multocida*)
  - Uterine or ovarian neoplasia
  - Uterine rupture
  - Any systemic disease causing lack of fitness or libido

STILLBIRTH, RESORPTION, ABORTION, CANNIBALISM AND DESERTION

These can easily be confused as parturition is rarely observed, and due dates often not known.

Stillbirth
- Hypo- and hypervitaminosis A
- Metritis
- Uterine torsion

Resorption
- Takes place before day 20
- Very common
- Peak incidence at approx 13 days (if doe is undernourished, obese, overcrowded or otherwise stressed)
- Another peak of fetal loss at approx 23 days (if doe is handled, causing physical dislodgement), due to temporary reduction in uterine blood flow as fetuses change size and shape

Abortion
- Takes place after day 24
- Relatively uncommon
- Listeriosis, *Salmonella infection*
- Pregnancy toxaemia

Cannibalism
- Environmental disturbance
- Disturbance of nest, doe or kits
- Overcrowding (by dam or other does)
- Primaparous or stressed does
- Over vigorous cleaning of newly born kits by naive does

Desertion
- Primaparous or stressed does

Be aware:
- Does normally suckle once (or occasionally twice) daily, for a few minutes only
- Does may not suckle young in the first 24 hours

Neonatal deaths
- Hydrocephalus and other congenital deformities
  - Due to hypo- and hypervitaminosis A
- Hypothermia
  - Kits leaving nesting area
  - Small or inadequately bedded nests
- Unhygienic nests due to does urinating and defecating in them
- Septicaemia or agalactia from staphylococcal mastitis
- Overfeeding of milk leading to faecal impaction around anus
  - Can lead to anal obstruction and gut stasis

Any or all of the above scenarios can occur due to:
- Short daylength
- Heat stress
- Concurrent systemic disease, e.g. *Salmonella*
- Uterine neoplasia
- Pregnancy toxaemia
- Obesity (increased resorption, abortion)
- *Treponema paraluis-cuniculi*
  - Can cause infertility, metritis, retained afterbirths, stillbirths and increased neonatal mortality

KEY HISTORY

- Age
- Sex
- Entire or neutered?
- Has this rabbit ever successfully given birth before this occasion?

- How long ago?
- Has oestrus behaviour been observed?
- Has the buck a proven history of recent fertility?
- Was there a dominant female rabbit present with this doe and the buck?
- Was mating behaviour observed? How often? (Around 85% of natural copulations are successful.)
- Has more than one buck been tried?
- Is there any history of recent or current disease in this or in contact rabbits?
- Have any other in-contact rabbits aborted?
- Are the siblings (and offspring) fertile?

PHYSICAL EXAMINATION

- Assess state of maturity and plane of nutrition
- Full clinical examination for any systemic disease
- Observe (directly or video) mating behaviour
- Abdominal palpation
- Examination of external genitalia
- Presence of any vaginal discharge or haematuria
- Presence of milk or cystic fluid discharge from nipples

DECISION-MAKING

- Is this rabbit already pregnant (possibly having delayed implantation)?
- Is the rabbit failing to become pregnant, or losing the fetuses?
- Is this an individual rabbit problem or a group problem?
- Assuming no intercurrent disease, would it be best to spay the rabbit? Or is breeding the primary purpose of this rabbit?
- Is this due to a behavioural problem, systemic disease or true infertility?

DIAGNOSTIC APPROACH

- Haematology and biochemistry
  - To diagnose intercurrent disease
  - Increased CK in vitamin E deficiency
- Work up any signs of intercurrent systemic disease as appropriate
- Fertilize by AI with semen from proven buck
- Hormonal induction of ovulation
  - Buserelin licensed in UK (Receptal®)
- Vaginoscopy
- Cytology from external genitalia and vagina

- Biopsy of any lesions
- Vaginal fungal and bacterial culture and sensitivity
- Abdominal radiography and ultrasonography
- Vagino-urethrogram
- Laparotomy to ensure presence and normality of ovaries and uterus, grossly and histopathologically
- Submit any aborted/stillborn fetuses, and placentas for culture and histopathology

INFERTILITY – MALE

As for General Infertility above, and also:
- Previous castration or vasectomy
- Paramphimosis following anaesthesia
- Genital tract disease
  - *Treponema paraluis-cuniculi*
  - Pasteurellosis
  - Testicular abscessation, orchitis and epididymitis (possible consequence of low grade myxomatosis)
  - Genital trauma
  - Congenital deformity
    — Cryptorchidism
    — Hypogonadia
    — Intersex
  - External genitalia trauma, inflammation, pain or deformity
  - Perineal pain, caecotroph accumulation, etc.
  - Fur accumulation around penis
- Systemic illness
  - Any systemic disease causing lack of fitness, libido or ability to mount doe, e.g. musculoskeletal disease
- Sperm defects
  - Inadequate numbers (inherent or over use)
  - Reduced motility (absolute or directional)
  - Morphological defects

- Insufficient stimulation to induce ovulation
  - Especially in bucks that are trained to use an artificial vagina

KEY HISTORY

- Age
- Neutered, vasectomized or entire?
- Has the buck successfully fertilized (other) does before?
- Has the buck been observed to successfully mate with the doe?
- Any signs of systemic disease?
- Any dysuria, haematuria, penile discharge or excessive cleaning of genital region?
- Any history or evidence of trauma?
- Has the buck been used with too many does or too often (1 buck to up to 30 does)

PHYSICAL EXAMINATION

- Full clinical examination for concurrent systemic disease
- Both testicles present in scrotum? (May require sedation to avoid retraction into abdomen.)

DIFFERENTIAL DIAGNOSIS

- If not, localization of absent testicle
  - True cryptorchids usually lack the scrotal sac on the affected side
- Examination of external genitalia and face
  - Star shaped scrotal scars suggestive of previous *Treponema paraluis-cuniculi* infection
- Examination of musculoskeletal system, in particular of hindlimb mobility

DECISION-MAKING

- Is this due to a behavioural problem, systemic disease or true infertility?
- Assuming no systemic disease, would it be best to castrate or retire the rabbit, or is breeding the primary purpose of the buck?

DIAGNOSTIC APPROACH

- Observe (directly or via video) mating behaviour
  - *NB*: rabbit copulation lasts only a few seconds and usually ends with the male falling off the female. This is normal.

- If behaviourally compatible and physically capable of mating, examine further for causes of true infertility
  - Examination of sperm sample, to include pH, volume, sperm numbers, sperm motility, sperm morphology, microbiology
- If unable to mate, examine further for signs of musculoskeletal/neurological/neuromuscular disease or genital disease
- In both cases, examine further for signs of systemic disease reducing either libido or fertility
- Palpation of testes, ultrasound examination, testicular biopsy
- Cytology of preputial fluid
- Cytology of external genital skin/fur and any skin lesions elsewhere (*Treponema paraluis-cuniculi*)
- Biopsy, impression smear, scraping or flushing of lesions
- Immediate examination using Giemsa stain or dark field and oil immersion microscopy
- Trial treatment for *Treponema paraluis-cuniculi* if suspicious lesions present

JAUNDICE (ICTERUS)

Icterus is a moderately uncommon presenting sign in the rabbit. Biliverdin is the predominant bile pigment in rabbits (around 70%); rabbits produce low but measurable levels of bilirubin. The majority of biliverdin is excreted and normal serum levels are very low. Biliverdin assays are not commercially available. Only some biliverdin is reduced to bilirubin, due to low levels of biliverdin reductase, and increased bilirubin can be seen in cases of cholestasis, particularly biliary tree obstruction by neoplastic masses or hepatic coccidiosis, and occasionally with anorexia (possibly due to decreased secretion, but possibly as an indicator of lipidotic swelling). Serum bilirubin levels

therefore reflect both hepatocellular function and biliary tree patency.

Use of 'Oxyglobin' can lead to apparent icterus, discoloured urine, and interference with blood parameters using some analysers.

CAUSES

Pre-hepatic

Production of bilirubin at a faster rate than it can be conjugated.

- Haemolysis
  - Haemolytic anaemia
  - Bacteraemia, septicaemia

- DIC/VHD
- Kale (in great excess), potato leaves and stems, and bracken can cause haemolysis

Hepatic

Decreased hepatic uptake and conjugation of bilirubin.

- Hepatic coccidiosis
- Hepatic lipidosis
- Hepatic neoplasia
- Liver fluke
- Toxic liver damage
  - Aflatoxins
  - Lead
  - Nitrophol agrochemicals
  - Drug induced
- Hepatic abscessation
- Hepatic fibrosis
- Liver lobe torsion
- Tyzzer's disease
- VHD
- Other less common causes
  - Hepatitis due to spread of intestinal infection via portal vein
  - Salmonellosis
  - Colibacillosis
  - Listeriosis
  - Toxoplasmosis
  - Tuberculosis
  - Tularaemia
  - Yersiniosis

Extra-hepatic

- Biliary tree obstruction
  - Hepatic lipidosis
  - Hepatic coccidiosis
  - Traumatic or abscess-related rupture of gall bladder/bile duct
  - Neoplasia

KEY HISTORY

- Age
- Sex
- Neutered or entire?

- Recent trauma or extreme physical exertion
- Recent drug or toxin exposure
- Condition of food supplies
- Deep litter, mesh floored or other substrate
- Behavioural changes, changes in activity, signs of abdominal pain
- Any other clinical signs
  - Anorexia
  - Weight loss/failure to grow
  - Diarrhoea
  - Abdominal distension
  - Death of in-contact animals
  - Abortion
- Depression
- Convulsions
- Other neurological signs
- Haemorrhage from orifices
- Respiratory signs
- Melaena
- Haemoglobinuria

PHYSICAL EXAMINATION

- Confirm presence of icterus
- Does rabbit appear anaemic also?
- Petechiation or ecchymosis
- Abdominal palpation and percussion
  - Hepatomegaly
  - Ascites
  - Uterine palpation
  - Abdominal pain (especially uterine)
- Auscultation of thorax and abdomen
- Pyrexia
- Hydration status
- Haematuria

DECISION-MAKING

- Is this true icterus (recent use of oxyglobin)?
- Is this likely to be due to current medication?
- Is the icterus pre-hepatic, hepatic or post-hepatic?

- Is this due to end stage hepatic lipidosis secondary to some other condition?

DIAGNOSTIC APPROACH

- Full haematology
- Clotting times
- Full biochemistry including bile acids (consider also BSP and ICG dye clearance)
- Urinalysis: haematuria, haemaoglobinuria
- Abdominal imaging: radiography and ultrasonography
- Faecal analysis: parasite oocysts, bacterial culture

- Peritoneal tap +/− abdominal lavage in cases of suspected ascites
- Laparotomy or laparoscopy
- Liver biopsy at laparoscopy/laparotomy/ ultrasound guided
- Biopsy evaluation
  - ○ Impression smear
  - ○ Cytology
  - ○ Histopathology
- Bacterial culture and sensitivity
- Calicivirus isolation/PCR
  - ○ Usually at post mortem or for groups of rabbits
- Culture of mouldy food for *Aspergillus* spp. or other fungal growth

KIT DISEASES AND FAILURE TO GROW

Normal development is variable with breed.
- Born naked and with eyes closed
- Doe attends the nest and feeds the kits for only 5 minutes once (or occasionally twice) a day
- Day 7, fur begins to grow
- Day 10, eyes open
- Day 12, ears open
- Day 18, venture from nest and start tasting food
- Day 35–60, fully weaned and independent

Congenital abnormalities
May be evident at birth or become clinically evident later in life
- Hydrocephalus and spina bifida due to hypo- or hypervitaminosis A
- Splay leg
- Eyelid defects
- Hereditary incisor malocclusion
- Collagen defects

First few weeks (pre-weaning)
(See also Cannibalism, Desertion and Neonatal deaths in Infertility – Female, pp. 43–44)

- Inexperienced doe
- Diseases of the doe affecting behaviour or lactation
- Staphylococcosis
  - ○ Ventral moist dermatitis at 10 days of age or less
  - ○ Conjunctivitis and multiple dermal abscesses 2–4 weeks
- Coliform diarrhoea
  - ○ Particularly a problem when attempting hand rearing of orphaned kits

During weaning (3.5–6 weeks of age)
- Viral (rotavirus) and bacterial (*Escherichia coli*, *Salmonella*) diarrhoea

Post-weaning (5–12 weeks of age)
- Coccidiosis
  - ○ Intestinal
  - ○ Hepatic
- Mucoid enteropathy syndrome
  - ○ Dysautonomia
  - ○ Rabbit epizootic enteritis

LYMPHADENOPATHY

Peripheral lymphadenopathy is a rare presenting sign in rabbits. Even cases with severe and chronic inflammatory disease, such as mandibular abscessation or pododermatitis, often do not have appreciable enlargement of the draining lymph nodes.

The predominant differential for enlargement of a lymph node is neoplastic disease, either within the peripheral area which drains to that lymph node, or more often as a consequence of lymphoma/lymphosarcoma – although even here abnormalities of internal lymphoid structures such as thymus (which normally persists throughout adulthood), mediastinal and mesenteric lymph nodes and bone marrow are more common.

KEY HISTORY

- Previous history of inflammatory or neoplastic disease
- Duration of enlarged lymph nodes
- Concurrent clinical signs
  - Anorexia
  - Weight loss
  - Dyspnoea
  - Weakness/collapse
  - Pallor
  - Exophthalmos

PHYSICAL EXAMINATION

- Single or multiple enlarged lymph nodes
- Evidence of concurrent infected or inflammatory lesions
- Evidence of visceral lymphadenopathy, thymic enlargement or bone marrow suppression

DECISION-MAKING

- Has an associated infected or inflammatory lesion been identified?

DIAGNOSTIC APPROACH

- Haematology
  - Particularly lymphocyte and other leucocyte morphology
- Fine needle aspirate cytology of affected node(s)
- Trucut biopsy (under local anaesthesia) of affected node(s)
- Thoracic +/– abdominal survey radiography
- Excisional biopsy of an entire lymph node
- Bone marrow aspiration

MYIASIS (FLYSTRIKE)

Myiasis (flystrike) is a common, distressing condition. The rabbit may be suffering pre-existing disease, and may be suffering the effects of shock as a result of its lesions. Flies do not attack normal rabbit skin. The skin must be damp, soiled, inflamed, etc., to attract flies. There is normally an underlying cause. Although not a true 'internal medicine' presentation, myiasis is included in this book because of the many medical predisposing causes.

TREATING FLYSTRIKE

- Stabilize rabbit
- Remove maggots
- Wound management
- Investigate underlying cause of flystrike
- Prevention of future attacks

Stabilize rabbit
- Wound itself is usually remarkably clean

DIFFERENTIAL DIAGNOSIS

- Main danger is shock
  - Fluid losses (flystrike akin to thermal burns)
  - Endotoxic shock from tissue damage
  - Pain and stress
- Antibiotics
- Aggressive fluid therapy
- Steroids or NSAIDs
  - Analgesia and anti-endotoxic shock treatment
- Further analgesia, e.g. opioids

Remove maggots
- Clip fur to examine more easily
- Rinse/wash fur and skin
- Physical removal by hand
- Warm air may draw maggots to surface
  - Hairdryer
- Water to flush out of pockets
  - Syringe
  - Dental machine
  - Ear cleaning flushing units
- Flush orifices/cavities with tubing introduced proximal to (deep to) maggots
- Larvicidal therapy. The following products have anecdotally been suggested, with varying effectiveness, to kill maggots present in tissues:
  - Avermectins
    — Ivermectin
    — Selamectin
  - Capstar
    — Nitenpyram (Novartis Animal Health)

Wound management
- Wounds rarely benefit from suturing
- Wounds usually very clean
  - Maggots eat necrotic tissue
  - Sterile maggots are used in human and veterinary medicine as debriding agents!
- May need edges debriding
- Systemic antibiotics

- Topical medications to promote healing, e.g. Dermisol (Pfizer), Flamazine (Smith-Nephew), Intrasite (Smith-Nephew), Nu-gel (Johnson and Johnson), Manuka Honey

Investigate underlying cause
- Diarrhoea
- Caecotroph accumulation
- Dermatitis
  - Contact irritancy
  - Atopy
- Myxomatosis
- Urine scalding
  - Incontinence
  - PU/PD
  - Inability to posture for urination
- Inguinal scent gland impaction
- Vaginal discharge
  - Pyometra
  - Post-partum
  - Intact females at increased risk generally over-spayed females
- Inability to clean area properly
  - Mobility problems
    — Spinal stiffness
    — Abdominal pain
  - Dental disease

Prevention
- Identification and treatment of underlying cause
- Deterrence of flies
  - Insect deterrents nearby
    — Local insect repellents
  - UV/electrocution grids
  - Mosquito netting
- Insect growth hormone regulators
  - Cyromazine (Rearguard®, Novartis Animal Health)
- Regular (twice daily) inspection of underside of rabbit

DIFFERENTIAL DIAGNOSIS

OBESITY, DIET AND EXERCISE

OBESITY

A lack of sufficient exercise +/− an excess of ingested calories, can result in obesity. This can affect the rabbit directly by making it physically difficult to ingest caecotrophs, and can lead to an excessively large dewlap or perineal skin fold formation, both of which further hinder ingestion; the latter predisposes to both urine scald and skin fold dermatitis.

Problems associated with obesity can include:

- Caecotroph accumulation
- Inability to groom properly
- Urine scald
- Myiasis (see p. 49)
- Increased incidence of clinically evident ectoparasitism
- Atherosclerosis
- Pododermatitis
- Musculoskeletal disorders
- Heat stroke and sudden death
- Hepatic lipidosis following pregnancy, sudden weight loss or inappetance

DIET

The 'natural' diet of the wild rabbit (*Oryctolagus cuniculus*) consists of large quantities of high fibre food (e.g. grass) eaten nearly continuously throughout the day, with caecotrophs ingested at times of the day when the rabbit is underground. In captivity, a typical diet often involves feeding a pelleted diet or cereal based 'rabbit mix', usually offered vastly in excess of nutritional requirements, with minimal provision of foodstuffs high in long indigestible fibre.

Physiologically, rabbits need to consume a diet containing indigestible fibre particles more than 0.5 mm in length for colonic motility to function effectively. Indigestible components are separated out and passed as 'hard faeces' and fermentable components are passed to the caecum where microbial action converts them into volatile fatty acids and microbial proteins which are then reingested as caecotrophs, and absorbed. Both indigestible fibre (the former) and fermentable fibre (the latter) are required. There is also an important role of both fibrous materials and calcium (and vitamin D when dietary calcium levels are low) in the diet in the prevention of dental disease.

A more naturalistic and nutritionally suitable approach therefore consists of feeding predominantly grasses (fresh or dried), hays, and fibrous leafy vegetables with a high calcium content (dark green leafy vegetables) ad libitum. To this basic diet, small amounts of root vegetables, fibrous fruits, and teaspoon quantities of pelleted diets can be added, particularly in the case of growing, pregnant or lactating individuals.

Problems associated with incorrect dietary intake are legion, but can include the following, either directly or indirectly:

- Obesity
- GI disorders
  - Reduced GI motility
  - Caecotroph accumulation
  - Diarrhoea
- Dental disease
- Urolithiasis
- Nutritional secondary hyperparathyroidism

EXERCISE

Guidelines for absolute minimum size of rabbit housing

- Horizontal − adequate space to achieve three 'hops' in a straight line
  - Equivalent to 2 metres for a NZW rabbit

- Vertical – sufficient to stand on hindlegs and stretch upwards fully unhindered

Problems associated with insufficient physical activity may include the following:
- Obesity
- GI disorders
  - Reduced GI motility

— the stomach in particular lacks much intrinsic motility, and depends partly on external movement of the rabbit
- Disuse atrophy of bony tissues
  - especially the vertebral column, contributing to lumbar fractures
- Subsequent urine scalding, flystrike or hindlimb paresis

PARESIS AND PARALYSIS

- Paresis – weakness of one or multiple areas of the body (mono, quadri, para, hemi)
- Plegia – paralysis, total loss of use of the area(s) (mono, quadri, para, hemi)

- Trauma
  - Spinal fracture or subluxation
- Spinal neoplasia

Quadriparesis/plegia
Difficult to differentiate true neurological quadriparesis from generalized weakness due to systemic disease.
- Congenital spinal abnormality
  - Hemivertebra (usually asymptomatic)
- Disc disease
  - Prolapse
  - Discospondylitis
- Infectious
  - Encephalitozoonosis
  - Spinal abscess
  - Toxoplasmosis
  - Listeriosis
  - Encephalitis
- Trauma
  - Spinal fracture or subluxation
  - Cranial trauma, concussion
- Spinal neoplasia
- Idiopathic
  - 'Floppy rabbit syndrome'

CAUSES

- Damage to the spinal cord or motor areas of the brain
  - Traumatic
  - Vascular
  - Inflammatory
  - Neoplastic
  - Compressive

Monoparesis/plegia
- Lateralized spinal damage
- Lower motor neuronal damage

Hemiparesis/plegia
- Rare
- Lateralized cervical spinal disease or intracranial lesion

Paraparesis/plegia
- Congenital spinal abnormality
  - Hemivertebra (usually asymptomatic)
- Disc disease
  - Prolapse
  - Discospondylitis
- Infectious
  - Encephalitozoonosis
  - Spinal abscess
  - Toxoplasmosis

KEY HISTORY

- Diet
  - Nutritional secondary hyperparathyroidism can predispose to spinal fractures
  - Nutritional muscular dystrophy
- Husbandry

- ○ Potential trauma
- ○ Predator attack
- ○ Access to toxins
- Acute onset or gradually progressive
- Weight loss or muscle wastage
- Signs of concurrent disease
  - ○ Pain – behaviour changes or pain response when touched
  - ○ Anorexia
- Other neurological signs
  - ○ History of seizures
  - ○ Collapse
  - ○ Tremors
  - ○ Head tilt
  - ○ Behaviour changes
- Urinary incontinence?

PHYSICAL EXAMINATION

Neurological examination of rabbits is frequently difficult due to the natural inclination of this prey species to freeze when in a stressful situation, and due to the natural flexed posture of the hindlimbs when 'standing'. Physical examination should particularly look for evidence of underlying systemic disease, and where possible should attempt to localize any neurological lesion.

DECISION-MAKING

- Primary neurologic disease or generalized weakness due to other primary cause?
- Localizable site of neurological lesion?
- Painful lesion?
- Likelihood of successful outcome?
  - ○ Lumbar spinal fracture is a common cause of hindlimb paresis and carries a very poor prognosis

DIAGNOSTIC APPROACH

Dependent on findings in clinical examination, but may include:
- Haematology and biochemistry (to rule out systemic disease)
- Serology (particularly *Encephalitozoon cuniculi*)
- Urinalysis (particularly trichrome stained cytology to look for *Encephalitozoon cuniculi*)
- Radiography (plain and myelogram where indicated)
- CSF analysis (may confirm presence of inflammatory lesion)
- MRI or CT

PODODERMATITIS

This can range from mild inflammation of the hocks, through to displacement of the superficial digital flexor tendon (perpetuating and worsening the problem), and deep ulcerative lesions with secondary infection, sometimes involving bone. Although not a true 'internal medicine' presentation, pododermatitis is included in this book because of the many medical predisposing causes.

PREDISPOSING FACTORS

- Poor anatomical conformation

- ○ Large rabbits
  - — Giant breeds
  - — Obesity
- ○ Lack of guard hairs
  - — Rex breeds
  - — Clipping of feet for surgery
- Husbandry problems
  - ○ Thumping with hind feet due to disturbance
  - ○ Inappropriate substrates, such as hard or abrasive surfaces, or wire mesh
  - ○ Poor hygiene, damp and/or dirty bedding
- Urinary and/or faecal incontinence

- Loss of or lack of weight bearing of another limb
- Stress factors affecting immune competence
  - Chronic disease
- Lack of mobility
  - Small cage
  - other locomotor lesions, such as spondylosis, ataxia

The single most important factor is flooring construction and substrate, and wire mesh is the most likely to cause pododermatitis. Wire mesh does not allow the rabbit to adopt a normal digitigrade stance (a normal rabbit bears the weight on its toes), subsequently bringing the hock (which does not normally bear any weight) into contact with the floor.

EFFECTS

Pododermatitis, as a source of chronic pain, infection, inflammation, blood loss, etc., can affect the rabbit in many ways.
- Anaemia due to blood loss
- Pain leading to gut stasis, aggression, etc.
- Chronic inflammation leading to amyloidosis of kidneys
- Chronic infection leading to anaemia

Treatment is challenging, and not always successful. Management of the underlying causes, use of NSAIDs, antibiotics, tissue repair promoting substances and strategic dressing of the feet, may all be necessary. Topical products such as Dermisol Cream (Pfizer Ltd), Flamazine Cream (Silver Sulfadiazine, Smith and Nephew Ltd), Bactroban Cream (Mupirocin Calcium, Glaxo Smith-Kline), etc. may be useful.

POLYURIA/POLYDIPSIA

PU/PD is a moderately common presenting sign in the rabbit. It may be true PU/PD, behavioural, physiological, or apparent PU/PD due to problems associated with drinking. Hyperadrenocorticism and diabetes insipidus are not reported in the pet rabbit population.

Normal water consumption
Consumption can vary dramatically in normal rabbits.
- Between strains
  - Differences in renal physiology, depending on availability of water in their environment
- Between lifestages
  - Especially increased in pregnancy, lactation
- Depending on water content of food

Apparent water consumption of greater than 100 ml/kg/day
- 'Playing' with drinker nozzle
- Inability to use drinker correctly, wasting water
- Dysphagia
- Faulty water bottles or drinkers
- Drinkers positioned too low to drink from effectively
- Spillage from water bowls

Genuine consumption of greater than 100 ml/kg/day
Physiological polydipsia
- Lactation
- Low water content of food
- High salt content of food
- Inappetance
- Low ambient humidity

Pathological polydipsia

- Behavioural polydipsia
  - Pyschogenic polydipsia has been diagnosed by exclusion in laboratory NZW rabbits: causes may have included boredom
  - Medullary washout through behavioural polydipsia may occur
- Oral pain
  - Dental disease
- Iatrogenic
  - Diuretics
  - Glucocorticoids
- Systemic disease
- Renal failure
- GI pathology leading to diarrhoea
- Mucoid enteropathy
- Diabetes mellitus
- Hepatic disease
- Sepsis
- Cystitis
- Urinary tract calculi/sludge

KEY HISTORY

- Age
- Sex
- Neutered or entire?
- Pregnancy/pseudopregnancy/lactation status
- Diarrhoea or lack of faecal output
- Appetite
- Diet
- Weight loss
- How is water provided?
- Have drinkers been checked for faults?
- Any puddles of water under drinker/around bowl?
- Any recent dietary changes?
- Has method of water provision changed?
- Environmental changes (increased temperature, indoors vs. outdoors)
- Is the rabbit housed alone or with others?
  - Is it this rabbit that is drinking more?
- Recent drug or supplement use, e.g. aminoglycosides, vitamin D
- Changes in urination
- How much is the rabbit drinking?
- Any signs of concurrent disease?

PHYSICAL EXAMINATION

- General demeanour
- Full clinical examination, particularly oral examination
  - Will probably necessitate examination under GA
- Hydration status
- Abdominal palpation, percussion and auscultation
- Dermatological evidence of endocrinopathy
- Any evidence of infection, e.g. vaginal discharge
- Faecal staining due to diarrhoea

DECISION-MAKING

- Is this due to true polydipsia or is water being lost in other ways (other rabbits drinking it, wastage, etc.)?
- If due to true polydipsia, is there a physiological reason for this, e.g. dietary change, lactation?
- Is the rabbit systemically unwell?
- Is there dental disease?

DIAGNOSTIC APPROACH

- Haematology, biochemistry and electrolytes
- Full urinalysis including
  - Culture and sensitivity
  - Creatinine clearance
- Radiographic and ultrasound examination of abdomen
- Full oral examination, under sedation/general anaesthetic as necessary
- Oral and pharyngeal endoscopy
- Skull radiography
- Encephalitozoonosis serology

DIFFERENTIAL DIAGNOSIS

PTYALISM (HYPERSALIVATION)

Hypersalivation (pytalism) involves excessive saliva secretion. In *pseudoptyalism* a normal amount of saliva is produced but there is dribbling due to dysphagia or lip abnormalities. The majority of cases are due to dental pathology.

CAUSES

Facial nerve paralysis affecting tongue or lips

- Traumatic (including iatrogenic following facial surgery)
- Abscess involvement
- Tooth root involvement

Facial distortion affecting lip apposition

- Dental disease
- Aural disease
  - Inflammation around the tympanum area, causing retraction of the lip on the affected side
- Trauma (soft tissue or involving mandible/maxilla) (including iatrogenic)
- Abscess formation
- Neoplasia

Lip pain

- Incisor dental disease
- Myxomatosis
- *Treponema paraluis-cuniculi*
- Trauma (including iatrogenic following incisor dentistry)

Oral cavity disease

- Dental disease
- Glossitis/stomatitis
  - Tooth related
  - Caustic
  - Azotaemia related
  - Electrical burn
- Neoplasia

- Trauma to tongue, gum and buccal mucosa, including iatrogenic following dentistry
- Oral foreign body (food/stick impaction)
- Oral inflammation from plant toxins, e.g. arum, fresh buttercups, spurges

Pharyngo-oesophageal swallowing disorders

- Neoplasia
- Tonsillar inflammation/lymphadenopathy
- Pharyngitis
- Laryngeal granuloma
- Cervical neoplasia, lymphadenopathy or abscessation
- Thoracic abscess or neoplasia
- Oesophagitis
- Oesophageal stricture
- Oesophageal foreign body
- Oesophageal diverticulum or rupture

Fluid overspill from stomach

- GI stasis + PU/PD
  - Rare, usually agonal event
  - e.g. mucoid enteropathy

Toxins

- Triazine agrochemicals, e.g. on treated hay
- Plant toxins, e.g. holly, elder, lobelia, iris, lupin and rhododendron

Systemic disease

- Pregnancy toxaemia
- Myasthenia gravis
- Rabies
  - Not seen in the UK
  - Paralytic rabies may be seen in the USA, usually after contact with affected racoons
- Tetanus (theoretically possible but not recorded in practice)
- Botulism (experimentally induced, but not reported in practice)

- *Encephalitozoon cuniculi* (not a usual sign)
- Dysautonomia can cause dysphagia and hypersalivation

KEY HISTORY

- Age
- Breed
- Diet
- Duration, severity and progression of disease
- Appetite. Is the rabbit systemically well?
- Is this associated with head tilt, nystagmus or falling to one side?
- Is this rabbit kept alone?
- Any history or evidence of trauma?
- Any history of recent dentistry or surgery?

PHYSICAL EXAMINATION

- Full clinical examination
- Complete and thorough dental/oral examination under sedation/GA as necessary
- Neurological examination and observation of locomotion
- Palpation of head and neck

- Abdominal palpation, percussion and auscultation

DECISION-MAKING

- Is this truly saliva, rather than wetting of the dewlap with drinking water?
- Is this due to excessive saliva production, or inability to swallow?
- If there are dental abnormalities, do I need to anaesthetize this rabbit and complete my dental examination, or has conscious examination been sufficient to arrive at a hopeless prognosis?

DIAGNOSTIC APPROACH

- Full clinical examination
- Haematology, biochemistry, electrolytes, *Encephalitozoon cuniculi* serology
- Complete and thorough oral/dental examination under GA
- Oral/pharyngeal endoscopy
- Skull radiography
  - Lateral, both oblique lateral views, and DV
- Neck radiography
- Fluoroscopy of rabbit swallowing
- Cranial MRI

PYREXIA

In contrast to canine and feline medicine, pyrexia in rabbits is relatively uncommon. This fact, and a very thin rectal/colonic mucosa with potential susceptibility to iatrogenic damage, makes routine temperature measurement somewhat superfluous in a standard clinical examination.

Many conditions which in canine or feline cases would result in pyrexia, such as abscesses, bite wounds, periodontal infection and even osteomyelitis, do not result in pyrexia in the rabbit.

NORMAL RECTAL TEMPERATURE

- 38.5–40°C
- Temperatures above 40.6°C are abnormal
  - Heat stroke (most common reason)
  - Severe systemic infection (septicaemia or viraemia)

DIFFERENTIAL DIAGNOSIS

INVESTIGATION

Attempt to isolate infectious causes of severe pyrexia.
- Full clinical examination
- Haematology and biochemistry evaluation

Heat stroke diagnosis is largely based on history of high ambient temperature and exclusion of other abnormalities.

TREATMENT

Depends on primary cause.
- infectious conditions
  - Intensive fluid therapy
  - Antibacterial therapy
  - Antiviral therapy if herpes virus encephalitis is suspected
- Heat stroke
  - Ambient cooling, e.g. wetting of the ears, cold hairdryer
  - Intravenous fluids
  - Corticosteroid therapy to combat shock

REGURGITATION AND VOMITING

Vomiting and regurgitation are extremely rare presenting signs in the rabbit. The well developed cardiac sphincter of the rabbit stomach precludes true vomiting, although fluid regurgitation can occasionally occur. Extremely rare idiopathic vomiting has also been anecdotally reported.

DIFFERENTIAL DIAGNOSIS

Vomiting and regurgitation are diagnoses of exclusion, following elimination of dysphagia, hypersalivation, oropharyngeal abscessation and upper respiratory tract discharge.

CAUSES

- Regurgitation is usually due to near-terminal gastric fluid overflow following GI stasis.
- Fluid is more likely to exit via the nose, or to be inhaled into the trachea, than it is to be expelled via the mouth.
- The most common cause is mucoid enteropathy, although theoretically any outflow disorder, combined with polydipsia

or iatrogenic food and fluid overload, could cause it.
- Very rare cases involving rabbits in group situations who eat extremely quickly and almost immediately regurgitate their food have been reported anecdotally. This has only been reported in situations where rabbits are fed highly palatable items intermittently, rather than being fed an appropriate high fibre diet ad libitum.
- True vomiting is so rare as to be almost unheard of:
  - A very small number of cases have been anecdotally reported. Cause is unknown. Some have had multiple episodes, some time apart, which seem to respond to symptomatic treatment on each occasion.

KEY HISTORY

- History of previous episodes
- History of respiratory tract disease
- History of dental disease
- Is the rabbit group housed?
- Has the rabbit been observed to eat extremely rapidly?

- Has the rabbit actually been directly observed to 'vomit'?
- If so, could this be dysphagia?

DECISION-MAKING

- Is this really vomiting/regurgitation?
- Is this terminal fluid overflow from stomach?
  - If so, rabbit is likely to be *in extremis*

DIAGNOSTIC APPROACH

- Full clinical examination
- Abdominal palpation, percussion and auscultation
- Presence of diarrhoea, mucus or lack of faecal output along with fluid or gas in the GIT and a palpable turgid stomach supports diagnosis of GI stasis

- Microscopic examination of the material is advised to differentiate vomitus from nasal discharge; measurement of the pH of the fluid may also help in differentiating between gastric and non-gastric sources
- Observation (direct or video evidence) of 'vomiting'
- Radiography of thorax for evidence of inhalation pneumonia, supporting the diagnosis of vomiting or regurgitation; also for evidence of oesophageal disease or mediastinal disease, both of which could cause dysphagia
- Full oral examination for evidence of dysphagia
- Rhinoscopy for evidence of upper respiratory tract disease
- Oesophageal endoscopy
- Examination of medial carpi for presence of discharge or vomitus

SEIZURES

Seizure is defined as a sudden attack of central neurological disturbance, and can be divided into grand mal seizure, petit mal seizure and partial seizure.

Grand mal seizure
- Unconsciousness
- Generalized muscular activity
  - Locomotive movements of the limbs
  - Chewing activity
  - Opisthotonos
  - Hypersalivation
  - Urination
- There may be a brief period of restlessness before the seizure

Petit mal seizure
- A mild, brief, but generalized seizure

Partial seizure (focal seizure)
- Restricted to a single area of the brain, and therefore causing uncontrolled motor activity of isolated area or limb, or simply behavioural abnormalities or apparent blindness

CAUSES

- Idiopathic
  - Epileptiform seizures with no apparent cause
  - Occasionally seen in rabbits
  - More prevalent in blue-eyed white breeds
- Encephalitozoonosis
  - Inflammatory response to encysted encephalitozoon organisms can result in seizures either as a direct consequence of inflammation or as a

consequence of restriction to blood-flow to other areas of the brain
  o Other parasitic infestations, such as toxoplasmosis and aberrant ascarid migration, may occasionally cause seizures
- Infection of the brain or meninges
  o Bacterial (septicaemic)
  o *Listeria*
  o Herpes simplex virus (human)
- Arteriosclerosis
  o Mineralization of meningeal blood vessels
  o Embolic incident
- Space occupying intracranial lesions
  o Abscessation (most commonly extension of an otitis)
  o Neoplasia
- Hypoxia
  o Severe cardiorespiratory disease
- Metabolic disease
  o End stages of renal or hepatic failure (especially hepatic lipidosis)
- End-stage systemic disease
  o Terminal stages of:
    — Septicaemia
    — Toxaemia (ingested toxins such as lead, or endotoxaemia)
    — VHD

KEY HISTORY

- Breed
- History of seizures in parents or littermates
- Single or recurrent event

- Previous or concurrent disease history
- Speed of onset of seizure and recovery, pre/post ictal signs?

PHYSICAL EXAMINATION

Full physical and neurological examination, particularly to differentiate between primary neurological disease and neurological disease secondary to another (anorexia, infectious, toxic, respiratory) disease process.

DECISION-MAKING

- Are clinical signs of sufficient severity/duration to warrant euthanasia?
- Has the seizure finished or is it ongoing?
- Is stabilization therapy indicated?
  o Benzodiazepines
  o Intravenous fluid therapy
  o Barbiturates

DIAGNOSTIC APPROACH

- Haematology and biochemistry
- *Encephalitozoon cuniculi* serology
- Urine trichrome stained cytology (poorly sensitive but immediate test for *E. cuniculi*)
- Serum lead evaluation
- CSF analysis (particularly for signs of inflammatory disease)
- CT/MRI

SNEEZING AND NASAL DISCHARGE

CAUSES

Inhaled irritants

- Ammonia caused by poor hutch hygeine
- Dust from poor quality hay, straw, sawdust bedding
- Various household/DIY products
  - Shed/garage housed rabbits may be affected by petroleum products, creosote or paints
  - Indoor housed rabbits may be affected by air fresheners, disinfectants, perfumes or talcum powder

Foreign bodies

- Particularly pieces of hay which enter either nostril during feeding. Rabbits cannot visualize objects directly in front of the nose.

Infections

- Local
  - Rhinitis associated with *Pasteurella*, *Bordetella*, *Staphylococcus*
  - Mucocutaneous dermatosis associated with *Treponema cuniculi* infection
- Systemic
  - Pasteurellosis
  - Myxomatosis

Other causes

- Dacryocystitis and periodontal abscessation
- Neoplasia

KEY HISTORY

- Husbandry system, potential exposure to irritants
- Previous history of respiratory infection or dental disease
- Vaccination history
- Breeding history (potential exposure to syphilis?)
- Concurrent clinical signs

- Dyspnoea?
- Systemically unwell?
- Ocular discharge?
- Anorexia?
- Perineal lesions?
- Duration of clinical signs
- Is there sneezing, nasal discharge, or both?
- Unilateral vs. bilateral discharge

PHYSICAL EXAMINATION

- Examination of the nostrils and perinasal area. Also check for discharges on the inner aspects of carpi.
- Unilateral vs. bilateral discharge
- Nature of discharge
  - Serous
  - Mucoid
  - Purulent
- Evidence of systemic disease
- Evidence of dental disease
- Evidence of perineal dermatitis

DIAGNOSTIC APPROACH

- Unilateral
  - Radiography for tooth root lesions or tearduct obstruction
  - Endoscopic examination of the nasal cavity and pharynx +/– biopsy of gross lesions for histopathology
  - Nasal flushing
- Bilateral
  - Radiography for tooth root lesions or tearduct obstructions
  - Deep nasal swab for bacteriology (1–3 cm inside the nasal cavity; expect bleeding)
- Systemic/multifocal
  - Biochemistry and haematology
  - Additional bacteriology samples from conjunctiva
  - Biopsy and silver staining of nasal/venereal lesions for *Treponema*

STIFFNESS

Stiffness is an abnormality of locomotion or posture manifested as a restriction of movement or difficulty or reluctance to rise from recumbent position.

CAUSES

- Degenerative joint disease
- Infectious (septic) joint disease
- Spinal or abdominal pain
- Pododermatitis
- Encephalitozoonosis

KEY HISTORY

- Age, breed
  - Clinical degenerative joint disease is more common in older rabbits and giant breeds
- Husbandry
  - Likelihood of trauma
  - Predisposing factors for pododermatitis
- Onset
  - Acute vs. chronic
  - Progressive?
- Overt signs of pain at rest or when handled
- Signs of concurrent systemic disease
  - Anorexia
  - Altered production of faeces and urine
- Generalized or localized stiffness, persistent or intermittent?

PHYSICAL EXAMINATION

- Full clinical examination for signs of concurrent systemic disease
- Palpation of limbs, and especially joints, for swelling, heat, pain, crepitus
- Abdominal palpation
- Neurological examination and evaluation of muscle tone (can be difficult or even impossible in a rabbit)

DECISION-MAKING

- Musculoskeletal or systemic?
- Muscular, neurological or joint associated?
- Traumatic?

DIAGNOSTIC APPROACH

- Biochemistry, haematology, urinalysis to rule out systemic disease
- Radiography of joints and spine
- Arthrocentesis for cytology for bacteriological culture

STUPOR

Stupor involves a reduced level of consciousness and/or reduced responses to external stimuli. *Disorientation* involves inappropriate responses to external stimuli.

CAUSES

- CNS disease
  - Encephalitozoonosis
  - Cranial trauma
  - Encephalitis
  - Intracranial neoplasia
- Metabolic disease
  - Uraemia
  - Hepatic encephalopathy
  - Hypoxaemia
  - Ketosis
  - Dehydration

- Anaemia
- Cardiac disease
- Heat stroke
- Toxins
  - Endotoxaemia
  - Lead
  - Lettuce
  - Plant toxins
- Infections
  - Encephalitozoonosis
  - Sepsis
  - VHD
- Idiopathic
  - 'Floppy rabbit syndrome'
  - Peri-ictal

KEY HISTORY

- Single affected animal or multiple cases?
- Acute vs. chronic onset
- Progressive?
- Husbandry
  - Likelihood of trauma
  - Access to toxins
  - Overheating
- Known access to new plant materials or to large quantities of lettuce
- History of seizures
- Signs of underlying systemic disease?

PHYSICAL EXAMINATION

- Evidence of trauma?
- Evidence of systemic disease?
- State of circulation
- Thoracic auscultation
- Neurological examination (often not possible in the rabbit because of tendency to freeze when stressed and because of naturally flexed nature of the hindlimbs when standing)

DECISION-MAKING

- History or likelihood of trauma?
- History or likelihood of intoxication?
- History or likelihood of hyperthermia?
- Severe systemic disease?
- Intracranial disease?

DIAGNOSTIC APPROACH

- Haematology, biochemistry and urinalysis
- Survey radiography of skull, thorax, abdomen
- Cardiac ultrasonography
- CSF analysis
- MRI or CT

SUDDEN DEATH

Causes of sudden death may be evident from clinical signs shortly before death, or from external appearance of the recently deceased rabbit, but in many cases a full post-mortem examination is required. Be aware that although the owner may not notice any prior abnormalities, apparent 'sudden death' in rabbits can simply be the end stage of a more chronic debilitating disease.

DIFFERENTIAL DIAGNOSES

- Acute renal failure
  - Very acute renal failure, oliguria and death
  - Renal enlargement may be seen at post mortem due to congestive heart failure
  - See Urinary tract disease, p. 150.
- Cardiomyopathy
  - See Cardiovascular disease, p. 91.

DIFFERENTIAL DIAGNOSIS

- *Encephalitozoon cuniculi*
  - Acute brain damage leading to seizure and death
  - Cardiac lesions.
- Electrocution
  - Rabbits commonly chew electrical wires, selectively stripping off the PVC coating
- Enterotoxaemia
  - See Diarrhoea, p. 19.
  - See Large intestinal disorders, p. 133.
- Heatstroke
  - In hot and especially humid, weather
- Haemorrhage
  - Internal, e.g. uterine endometrial venous aneurysm
  - See Disorders of the female genital tract and mammary glands, p. 168.
  - External, e.g. bite trauma, ulcerative pododermatitis
- Neoplasia
  - Rupture/haemorrhage, pulmonary involvement
- Listeriosis
- Intestinal obstruction
  - Acute abdomen
  - See Oesophageal disorders, p. 123 and Gastric disorders, p. 124.
  - See Small intestinal disorders, p. 131.
- Oesophageal obstruction (choke)
  - See Oesophageal disorders, p. 123 and Gastric disorders, p. 124.
- Severe respiratory tract lesion
  - Tracheal or laryngeal obstruction (foreign body, granuloma, neoplasm)
  - Fluid, infection (pasteurellosis, haemorrhage, etc., causing acute dyspnoea)
- Predator attack: traumatic or cardiac arrest
  - Traumatic injury to head, spine, neck or chest, depending on predator species
  - 'Night fright' not uncommon: attack or threat by predator leads to death from cardiac arrest, or through trauma after jumping into enclosure walls in attempt to flee
- Pregnancy toxaemia
  - Acute metabolic crisis and death
- Torsion of internal organ
  - Uterine torsion: see Disorders of the female genital tract and mammary glands, p. 168.
  - Liver lobe torsion: see Hepatobiliary tract disorders, p. 142.
- Rupture of abdominal mass, e.g. uterus, neoplasm
  - See Abdominal enlargement, p. 3.
  - See Ascites, p. 8.
  - See Disorders of the female genital tract and mammary glands, p. 168.
- Other trauma
  - Falls, ballistic injuries, crushing injuries
- Seizure
  - See Seizures, p. 59.
- Toxicity, e.g. plant, herbicide
  - See Nutritional requirements of rabbits, p. 105.
- Viral haemorrhagic disease
  - See Calicivirus infection, p. 177.

KEY HISTORY

- Time of day of death
- Indoor or outdoor rabbit
- Exposure to known or possible toxins
- Access to predators
- History of relevant disease, e.g. cardiac disease, dental disease
- History of deaths or disease in in-contact rabbits
- Recent weather and microclimate conditions
- VHD vaccination status
- Male, female, entire, neutered, pregnant or not
- History of access to potential intestinal foreign bodies

EXTERNAL PHYSICAL EXAMINATION

- General body condition.
- Signs of respiratory tract disease
  - Nasal discharge
  - Matting of hair on carpi
- Signs of predation (wounds on neck, head and chest)
- Signs of bleeding from orifices (mouth, nares, genitals, anus)
- Signs of other internal bleeding
  - Joint swelling
  - Petechial haemorrhages
  - Distended abdomen
- Signs of electrocution
  - Burns, especially on mouth or feet
  - Damage to wiring to which rabbit has access
- Signs of dental disease

POST-MORTEM EXAMINATION

A full discussion of post-mortem technique is outside the remit of this text. A comprehensive discussion on post-mortem examination can be found in *Textbook of Rabbit Medicine* (Harcourt-Brown, 2002a).

The following should be examined in particular:

- Skin of the neck for small puncture wounds
  - Predation
- Oropharyngeal cavity
  - Foreign body in larynx
  - Laryngeal granuloma

- Oesophagus
  - Foreign body
- GIT (especially points at which foreign body impaction are common)
  - Foreign bodies
  - Stomach contents for toxic plants
  - Signs of acute enteritis
- Abdominal cavity
  - Inspection of liver for signs of VHD
  - Examination of any organs that may have ruptured or haemorrhaged
  - Examination of uterus for pregnancy
- Thoracic cavity
  - Inspection for fluid, hemorrhage or space occupying lesion
  - Examination of lungs, heart and great vessels
- Examination of brain
  - Gross examination and collection of samples for histopathology

FURTHER EXAMINATION

- Toxicology
  - From gut contents, liver or kidney
  - Discussion with the diagnostic laboratory is advised before taking samples for toxicology
- Radiology
  - Survey radiographs for signs of trauma, cervical dislocation or ballistic injury
- Histopathology
  - Histopathology of any abnormal tissue
  - Histopathology of liver, lung, heart, brain, kidney

DIFFERENTIAL DIAGNOSIS

TREMOR

Tremor is defined as involuntary repetitive rhythmic muscle fasciculations.

NB: It is normal for there to be regular twitching of the upper lip and nose area of a rabbit – absence of this rhythmic twitching can be a sign of pain. It is also normal for rabbits to develop a tremor of the limbs, particularly the forelimbs when restrained in dorsal recumbency (or when hypnotized/tranced). Tremors are otherwise a rare presenting sign in the rabbit.

CAUSES

- Encephalitozoonosis
- Metabolic disease
  - Hepatic encephalopathy
  - Hypocalcaemia
  - Hypoglycaemia
  - Uraemia
- Paresis
- Systemic illness
- Lead or organophosphate toxicity
- Intracranial neoplasia
- Inherited

KEY HISTORY

- Age at onset
  - ? Hereditary causes or *in utero* brainstem damage if present from birth
- Health of littermates
- Diet
- Husbandry
  - Possible exposure to toxins or trauma

- Speed of onset, duration and progression
- Continuous or intermittent
- Behavioural changes or altered mental state

PHYSICAL EXAMINATION

Aim to rule out systemic disease, metabolic and toxic causes
- Mental status
- Evidence of pain
- Neurological examination. However, this is often not possible in rabbits because of a tendency to freeze when animal is stressed, and because of the naturally flexed state of hindlimbs when standing.

DECISION-MAKING

- Congenital or acquired?
- Underlying systemic disease?
- Other neurologic disturbance?

DIAGNOSTIC APPROACH

- Haematology and biochemistry
- *Encephalitozoon cuniculi* serology
- Urinalysis, particularly trichrome stained cytology to look for *E. cuniculi*
- Survey radiography
- CSF analysis (for evidence of inflammatory brainstem disease)
- MRI or CT
- EEG, EMG

WEIGHT LOSS

Weight loss is one of the most common presenting signs in rabbits. There are a large number of differential diagnoses, and it is perfectly possible for more than one factor to be involved at once.

CAUSES

Anorexia (see Anorexia, p. 6)
Inability to prehend food (see Dysphagia, p. 25)
- Neurological causes
- Musculoskeletal causes
- Dental causes

Inappetance
- Oral causes
  - Dental
  - Oral soft tissue
  - Foreign body in mouth or oesophagus

Further GIT problems
- Intestinal hypomotility
- Parasitism
  - Intestinal coccidiosis
  - *Cryptosporidium*
  - Stomach worm infestation
  - Pinworm (*Passalurus* spp.). Even in large numbers this worm is not usually associated with pathology or weight loss

Other reasons for inappetance
- Pain, stress, etc.
- Any environmental change
- Inappropriate food presented to rabbit
- Drug/vaccine induced anorexia
- Water deprivation
- Systemic disease
  - Any chronic inflammatory disease
  - Hepatic disease
  - Renal failure
  - Neoplasia
  - Pyrexia

- Soft tissue mineralization
- Cardiac disease
- Respiratory tract disease
- Rhinitis – any condition affecting the rabbit's sense of smell will adversely affect appetite
- Lower respiratory tract disease

Infectious disease
- Pasteurellosis
- Myxomatosis
- VHD
- Yersiniosis (pseudotuberculosis)
- Johne's disease (paratuberculosis)
- Tyzzer's disease
- *Encephalitozoon cuniculi*
- *Treponema paraluis-cuniculi*

Toxicity
- Lead poisoning
- Agrochemicals, e.g. triazine in treated hay
- Plant toxins causing GI irritation
- Aflatoxicosis

Energy malnutrition
- Insufficient quantity of food presented
- Dominant rabbit(s) eating all food or preventing access to it
- Unpalatable or unfamiliar food offered

Endocrine causes of weight loss
- Diabetes mellitus

Absorption disorders
- Intestinal neoplasia
- Chronic inflammatory bowel disease
- Chronic Tyzzer's disease, pseudotuberculosis, etc.

Neoplasia
- Direct effects on gut, e.g. space occupying lesion/obstruction
- As a cause of discomfort
- Catabolic effects

DIFFERENTIAL DIAGNOSIS

Other catabolic conditions
- For example, cardiac disease

Protein losing conditions
- Nephropathies
- Enteropathies

Pregnancy and lactation
- Inadequate food input relative to energy expenditure

KEY HISTORY

- Age
- Sex
- Neutered or entire
- Diet
- Is the rabbit kept by itself?
- If with other rabbits, has this one been observed to be able to get to food?
- Could the rabbit be pregnant/lactating?
- Has there been any recent dietary change?
- Has the rabbit changed its dietary preferences?
- Has there been any change of water provision?
- Has there been any recent environmental change?
- Is the rabbit well in itself?
- Is the rabbit leaving any food?
- Has the rabbit been observed eating?
- Is there any nasal discharge or sneezing?
- Is there any epiphora or ocular discharge?
- What is the rabbit's vaccination status?
- Has the rabbit recently been given any drugs or vaccinations?
- Duration, severity and progression of weight loss?

- Have any in-contact rabbits had any clinical signs?
- Any changes in urination?
- Any changes in defecation?

PHYSICAL EXAMINATION

- Full clinical examination
- Thorough and complete oral examination
- Abdominal palpation, percussion and auscultation
- Examination of medial carpi for discharge
- Examination of nasolacrimal ducts for discharge
- Body temperature

DECISION-MAKING

- Is the rabbit getting enough to eat?
- Is the rabbit's appetite good?
- Is this due to dental disease or systemic disease?

DIAGNOSTIC APPROACH

- Full oral examination under sedation/GA
- Oral cavity endoscopy
- Skull radiography
- Haematology, biochemistry
- Skull CT scan
- Serology for *Encephalitozoon cuniculi*
- Abdominal and thoracic survey imaging
- Urinalysis for blood, sediment microscopy
- ECG
- Cardiac ultrasonography
- Bone marrow biopsy

SECTION 2
COMMON LABORATORY ABNORMALITIES

FACTORS AFFECTING HAEMATOLOGICAL AND BIOCHEMICAL PARAMETERS

DIURNAL RHYTHMS

- Total white blood cell count
  - Lowest in the late afternoon/evening
- Lymphocyte count
  - Lowest in the late afternoon/evening
- Heterophil count
  - Highest in the late afternoon/evening
- Eosinophil count
  - Highest in the late afternoon/evening
- Cholesterol
  - Highest in the late afternoon/evening
- Urea
  - Highest in the late afternoon/evening

EFFECTS OF STRESS

- Prolonged stress (i.e. stress of disease, transport or unfamiliar surroundings, rather than handling alone) may result in heterophilia, lymphopaenia, increased blood glucose
- Chronic stress or disease may result in anaemia (decreased PCV, haemoglobin and RBC count)

PHYSICAL RESTRAINT

Increased
- Lactate dehydrogenase
- Aspartate aminotransferase
- Creatine kinase

HAEMOLYSIS

Increased
- Lactate dehydrogenase
- Aspartate aminotransferase
- Creatine kinase
- Total protein
- Potassium

Decreased
- Amylase

OXYGLOBIN

(Haemoglobin-based oxygen carrying solution, Biopure, USA)
- Can cause severe artefactual changes in some serum biochemistry results, depending on the methods used

ANAEMIA AND RED CELL CHANGES

Anaemia is a common finding in rabbits. This is less often due to blood loss than to non-regenerative anaemia for other reasons.

REGENERATIVE VS. NON-REGENERATIVE ANAEMIA

- Anisocytosis, polychromasia, nucleated RBCs and Howell–Jolly bodies can all be found in normal rabbit blood, in addition to being indicators of regenerative anaemia
- Heterophilia may be seen in haemolytic or haemorrhagic anaemia
- Significant, rapid reticulocyte production is seen in the healthy rabbit following blood loss

CAUSES OF REGENERATIVE ANAEMIA

Blood loss
- External
  - Wounds
  - Severe ectoparasitism
- Internal
  - Haematuria
  - Haematochezia
  - Endometrial venous aneurysm
  - Bleeding neoplasm
    — particularly uterine adenocarcinoma
  - Organ (liver, spleen) rupture following trauma

Ivermectin toxicity
- Rare
- Reduced RBC count, PCV, haemoglobin, MCV

Lead toxicosis
- Nucleated RBCs
- Poikilocytosis
- Hypochromasia
- Basophilic cytoplasmic stippling

Bleeding disorders
Blood sampling (especially in smaller rabbits) can be problematic, and contamination of blood with tissue fluids, or slow withdrawal of blood before contact with anticoagulant can lead to activation of clotting mechanisms and invalidation of results. A diagnosis of coagulopathy should only be arrived at if these factors are negated.

- Inherited disorders
  - Autosomal bleeding disorder similar to von Willebrands
    — inbred strain of Flemish Giant–Chinchilla crossbred rabbits
  - Haemophilia
    — Belgian hares
  - Autosomal recessive haemolytic anaemia

- Toxic disorders
  - Endotoxin exposure
    — DIC
  - Kale, leaves and stems of potato plants
    — Haemolytic anaemia
  - Alliums (onions, garlic and chives)
    — Heinz body anaemia
    — Susceptibility varies with species
    — Rabbits do not appear to be especially susceptible
- Paraneoplastic
  - Haemolytic anaemia in rabbits with thymoma and lymphosarcoma
- Iatrogenic
  - Thrombocytopaenia and coagulopathy is seen in excessive lipid administration using parenteral nutrition

CAUSES OF NON-REGENERATIVE ANAEMIA

Toxins
- Bracken ingestion causes bone marrow suppression in other herbivores

Chronic disease
- Otitis media
- Abscess
- Endometritis/pyometra/uterine adenocarcinoma
- Pneumonia
- Mastitis
- Bacterial cellulitis
- Pododermatitis
- Osteomyelitis
- Septicaemia
- Renal disease
- Lymphosarcoma (+/– bone marrow involvement)
- Dental disease (even without apparent infection)
- Chronic stress

Red cell changes other than anaemia

- Increased PCV
  - Dehydration, especially due to enteritis or gut hypomotility
- Nucleated RBC increase also seen with
  - Acute infection
  - Endothelial damage

WHITE BLOOD CELL CHANGES

- The healthy rabbit typically has a predominance of lymphocytes, with a ratio of approximately 40% heterophils to 60% lymphocytes
  - This state often reverses, with heterophil dominance occurring, in infectious disease
- Absolute leucocytosis is, however, rare
  - It can be seen in cases of lymphosarcoma
- In severe or chronic infections, toxaemia or viral infection, the total white cell numbers may decrease
- Band forms and a 'left shift' are not typically seen with infection
- Diurnal variation in total white blood cell counts
  - Highest in late afternoon/early evening
- Variation with age, being higher in rabbits of
  - 3 months (due to a lymphocyte peak)
  - 1 year (due to a heterophil peak)

HETEROPHILS

- Variable nomenclature
  - Sometimes called neutrophils, pseudo-eosinophils, acidophils or amphophils
- Analogous to (functionally identical to) the neutrophil in other mammals
- Larger cytoplasmic granules correspond to azurophilic granules of canine neutrophils
- Smaller granules correspond to the secondary granules in other mammals

Thrombocyte decrease

- Acute infection/septicaemia leads to decrease in numbers
- Clotted samples will falsely lower thrombocyte counts (see above)
- DIC
- Haemorrhage

Heterophilia

- Adrenocortical stress
- Exogenous glucocorticoids
- Acute infections, especially pyogenic bacteria
- Uterine and ovarian abscessation
- Autoimmune haemolytic anaemia

Heteropaenia

- Sepsis
- Toxaemia, e.g. uraemia

LYMPHOCYTES

- Large and small lymphocyte populations
- Usually the predominant WBC (up to 60%)

Lymphocytosis

- Viral infections may raise lymphocyte count
- Lymphoma

Lymphopaenia

- Adrenocortical stress
- Exogenous glucocorticoids
- Bacterial infections
- Dental disease
- Decrease with age

MONOCYTES

- Largest of the rabbit leucocytes

COMMON LABORATORY ABNORMALITIES

Monocytosis
- Chronic inflammation, abscessation
- Toxicity can lead to large dark red cytoplasmic granules

EOSINOPHILS

Eosinophilia
- Traumatic wound repair
- (Hypersensitivity induced eosinophilia is rare)
- Parasites migrating through tissues (but not *Encephalitozoon cuniculi*)
- Chronic suppurative disease or neoplasia (especially ovary and bone)
- Diseases of tissues containing mast cells, e.g. skin, GIT, uterus and lung

Eosinopaenia
- Adrenocortical stress
- Exogenous glucocortoids

- Low numbers or no eosinophils are not necessarily abnormal in rabbits

BASOPHILS
- More common in the rabbit than in other mammalian species
- Can be present at up to 30% in the normal rabbit

Basophilia (with concurrent eosinophilia)
- Atopy
- Chronic pyoderma
- Purulent inflammation of lung, skin, GIT or reproductive tract

Basophilia (without eosinophilia)
- Hyperlipoproteinaemia
- Primary liver disease
- Diabetes mellitus
- Nephrosis

AMYLASE AND LIPASE

AMYLASE

- Amylase is only produced by the pancreas in the rabbit, with little content in salivary glands or intestinal tissue
- None is produced by the liver
- Plasma half-life is 97 minutes (as opposed to 5 hours in the dog)

Causes of an increase in amylase
- Pancreatic damage (pancreatitis, pancreatic obstruction, abdominal trauma, peritonitis, neoplasia)
- Reduced clearance due to renal insufficiency

- Adrenocortical stress
- Glucocorticoid administration
- Reduced hepatic clearance

LIPASE

May be of use in determination of pancreatitis in the rabbit.

Causes of an increase in lipase
- Pancreatic damage
- Adrenocortical stress
- Glucocorticoid administration
- Reduced renal clearance

AZOTAEMIA

Azotaemia is:
- an increase of urea and creatinine above reference range
- not necessarily associated with clinical signs

Uraemia is:
- clinically significant azotaemia.

GENERAL COMMENTS

- Urea levels are inversely proportional to GFR, but urea is neither produced nor cleared at constant rates
- Serum levels depend on dietary and fermented protein levels, liver function, intestinal absorption, urease activity of the caecal flora and hydration status
- Recent feeding does not play a significant role as the stomach of the rabbit is rarely empty

Significant variations in urea levels can exist. They can be:
- Time related
  - Peak in late afternoon and early evening
- Breed related
  - Polish rabbits have higher levels than NZW or Dutch rabbits
  - NZW does have higher levels than bucks

Creatinine is a more reliable test of GFR.
- Old samples of blood (over 24 hours) can have artefactually low creatinine levels
- Elevated bilirubin can artefactually decrease creatinine levels
- Cephalosporins can artefactually increase creatinine levels

More direct methods include inulin clearance rate and endogenous/exogenous creatinine.

CAUSES OF AZOTAEMIA

Pre-renal
- Dehydration
  - Causes a rapid and surprisingly marked rise in urea and creatinine levels
  - Rapidly returns to normal once dehydration is corrected
  - Repeat sampling is necessary before a diagnosis of renal failure is made
- Decreased renal perfusion
  - Dehydration
  - Shock
  - Stress
  - Heat stroke
  - Water deprivation
  - Cardiac disease
- High protein diet
- GI haemorrhage
- Diarrhoea and weight loss increase nitrogen catabolism, increasing urea

Renal
- Renal parenchymal disease
- Nephrolithiasis
- Glomerular damage
- Acute or chronic renal failure

Post-renal
- Urinary tract obstruction
  - Uroliths
  - Sludge
  - UMN bladder
  - Neoplasia
  - Trauma
  - Bladder rupture
  - Urethral muscle spasm

COMMON LABORATORY ABNORMALITIES

Decreases in urea and creatinine

- Decreased urea can be a sign of excessive fluid throughput of non-renal origin, or of decreased hepatic function
- Decreased muscle mass (common in the end stages of dental disease) leads to decreased endogenous creatinine production

Elevations of urea and creatinine, once hydration status is normal, suggest losses of 50–70% of renal function, due to functional reserve capacity.

Urine relative density (SG) assists in differentiation between causes of azotaemia (see Urinalysis, p. 83 and Renal disease, p. 150).

ELECTROLYTE ABNORMALITIES

Electrolyte imbalances are common in rabbits due to their complex GI physiology, and large gut surface area, and the kidneys' limited ability to correct acid–base disturbances. Anorexia can lead rapidly to metabolic acidosis.

- Vitamin D is not important for uptake of calcium if dietary levels are high
  - It is important for absorption of calcium if dietary levels are low
  - It may play an important role in regulation of calcium distribution within the body

CALCIUM

The control mechanism for calcium metabolism in the adult rabbit is still not fully clear.

- In contrast to other mammalian species, calcium levels are much less tightly regulated
  - Blood calcium levels are far more significantly influenced by dietary levels than in the cat and dog
  - Rate of calcium excretion is related to dietary calcium intake
  - Urinary fractional excretion rate for calcium is in the order of 45–60%, as opposed to typical rates of 2% for other mammals
- A distinction between total (ionized + protein bound) calcium, and ionized calcium needs to be made
  - The latter gives a more accurate idea of the rabbit's metabolic state with respect to calcium
  - The former may give a more accurate picture of dietary intake and other metabolic parameters (pregnancy, serum protein levels, etc.)

TOTAL CALCIUM

Hypocalcaemia

- Halothane anaesthesia
- Diarrhoea
- Dietary insufficiency
- Hypoalbuminaemia
- Late pregnancy and lactation

Hypercalcaemia

- Excessive dietary intake
- Thymoma, and some other neoplasms, although not as commonly as in other species
- Renal disease (associated with clear urine)

IONIZED CALCIUM

Hypocalcaemia

- Halothane anaesthesia
- Diarrhoea
- Dietary insufficiency

Hypercalcaemia

- Excessive dietary intake

- Thymoma, and some other neoplasms, although not as commonly as in other species
- Renal disease

PHOSPHATE

Hyperphosphataemia
- Severe renal insufficiency
- Excessive dietary intake (oversupplementation)
- Intestinal disorders
- Haemolysis (true or artefactual)
- Soft tissue trauma
- Dehydration
- Bladder rupture

Hypophosphataemia
- Use of phosphate binders
- Reduced intestinal absorption
- Dietary deficiency

POTASSIUM

Potassium measurements are unreliable if taken through a plastic cannula.

Hyperkalaemia
- Renal failure
- Post-renal obstructions
- Severe tissue damage, especially crushing injuries
- Metabolic acidosis
- Artefactually, due to haemolysis or leakage from RBCs if not separated promptly

Hypokalaemia
- Anorexia/dietary lack
- Diuresis
- Metabolic alkalosis
- Loss of potassium rich fluid, e.g. saliva
- Polyuric renal failure

- Diarrhoea, especially with mucus secretion
- Catecholamine release following stress
- Artefactually with hyperproteinaemia or lipaemia

Hypokalaemia is a possible differential in 'floppy rabbit syndrome' (see Collapse/syncope, p. 16).

SODIUM

Hypernatraemia
- Loss of water of fluids low in sodium
  - Diarrhoea
  - Peritonitis
  - Burns, flystrike
- Water deprivation
- Excess salt in diet
- Prolonged exhaustion/exertion

Hyponatraemia
- Chronic renal failure
- Polyuric acute renal failure
- Nephritic syndrome
- Severe liver disease
- End stage CHF
- Diuretic use
- Artefactually with lipaemia or hyperproteinaemia

CHLORIDE

Hyperchloraemia
- Metabolic acidosis
  - Dehydration
  - Diarrhoea
  - Shock
- Renal failure, pyelonephritis
- Severe exhaustion or muscular exertion

Hypochloraemia
- Metabolic alkalosis
- Excessive diuresis
- Respiratory acidosis

COMMON LABORATORY ABNORMALITIES

CHOLESTEROL AND TRIGLYCERIDES

Levels peak after a meal, especially a fatty meal, in other species. In rabbits it is difficult to obtain a fasting sample due to caecotroph ingestion.

A lipaemic sample in anorexic rabbits indicates end stage hepatic lipidosis and problems with fat metabolism. These carry a poor prognosis.

CHOLESTEROL

- Normal levels of cholesterol vary dramatically between breeds of rabbit
  - Watanebe laboratory rabbits are bred specifically to be hypercholesterolaemic, even on low (zero) fat diets
- Males usually have lower cholesterol levels than females
- Cholesterol levels are higher in late afternoon/early evening

Elevated cholesterol
- Hepatic disease, especially hepatic lipidosis and bile stasis

- Raised endogenous or exogenous glucocorticoid administration
- Excessive dietary fat intake
- Pancreatitis
- Uterine abscessation
- Diabetes mellitus
- Nephrotic syndrome

Decreased cholesterol
- Chronic malnutrition
- Pregnancy (up to 30% lower in pregnancy)

TRIGLYCERIDES

Elevated triglycerides
- Diabetes mellitus
- Chronic renal failure
- Obesity
- Hepatic lipidosis

GLUCOSE ABNORMALITIES AND FRUCTOSAMINE

GLUCOSE

Stress is a *very* common reason for hyperglycaemia.
- Rabbits are easily stressed by handling, transport, presence of predators and strangers, venepuncture and the stress of underlying disease processes
- One-off raised blood glucose readings, however high, are insufficient for diagnosis of diabetes mellitus (DM), the frequency of which in rabbits is controversial, since rabbits rely much more on volatile fatty acid metabolism for their energy needs than on carbohydrates

- Although laboratory strains have been bred to develop DM, and the disease can be induced by pancreatic destruction, its existence in the pet rabbit population has not been proven
- Serial blood glucose levels, urinalysis and serum fructosamine, in conjunction with appropriate clinical signs, are necessary to arrive at such a diagnosis
- A true fasting sample is difficult to obtain, due to caecotrophy

Hyperglycaemia
- Stress
- Convulsions
- Shock

- Halothane anaesthesia
- Morphine or ketamine administration
- Hyperthermia
- Blood loss
- Early mucoid enteropathy
- DM
- Enteritis
- Glucose-containing parenteral fluids
- Renal insufficiency
- Drug therapy, especially glucocorticoids
- Hepatic lipidosis
- Intestinal foreign body or terminal gut stasis
  - Often severely raised
  - Poor prognostic sign

Hypoglycaemia
- Terminal anorexia
- Chronic debility
- Hepatic disease, especially hepatic lipidosis
- Sepsis
- Mucoid enteropathy
- Artefactually if sample not tested immediately or placed in fluoride oxalate tube soon after it has been taken

FRUCTOSAMINE

Fructosamine has been used as a marker for DM in the rabbit, and correlates much better than glucose with clinical signs of disease.

LIVER ENZYMES AND ASSOCIATED PARAMETERS

ALKALINE PHOSPHATASE (AP)

- Three separate isoenzymes
- None affected by handling or restraint
- Not liver specific
  - Also occur in osteoblasts, renal tubules, intestinal epithelium and placenta

Causes of an increase in AP
- Increases due to hepatic necrosis are negligible
  - Hepatic elevations are usually seen as a response to increased bile acids following bile stasis rather than hepatocellular damage
- Bile stasis
  - Hepatic lipidosis
  - Liver fluke
  - Hepatic coccidiosis
  - Liver abscessation, neoplasia
  - Extra-hepatic neoplasia, abscessation etc.
- Growth and bone lesions
- Artefactually increased with haemolysis

Decreases
- Diarrhoea
- Pregnancy

ALANINE AMINOTRANSFERASE (ALT)

- Not liver specific
- Also found in cardiac muscle and elsewhere
- An indicator of hepatocellular damage
- Increase does not correlate with degree of hepatic damage
- Sensitive but not specific

Causes of an increase in ALT
- Hepatocellular damage
- Hepatic lipidosis
- Neoplasia
- Anaesthesia
- Hepatic coccidiosis
- Use of pine or cedar shavings as litter substrate
- Aflatoxicosis

- Rabbits have lower tissue levels than carnivores
  - Approximately one-third of levels in the dog
  - Half-life of about 5 hours as opposed to 45 hours in the dog
- Artefactually increased with haemolysis

ASPARTATE AMINOTRANSFERASE (AST)

- Not liver specific
- Also occurs in cardiac and skeletal muscle, kidney and pancreas
- Highest levels in liver and skeletal muscle
- AST has a short half-life in the rabbit (around 5 hours)
- Compare with CK for meaningful interpretation (see Creatinine kinase, below)

Causes of an increase in AST

- Hepatocellular necrosis
- Hepatic coccidiosis
- Skeletal muscle damage or catabolism
  - Levels rise after restraint due to skeletal muscle damage
- Cardiac ischaemia
- Artefactual increases seen with haemolysis and increased bilirubin

GAMMA-GLUTAMYL TRANSFERASE (GGT)

- The most liver specific of the enzymes. GGT is also found in the kidney, but renal GGT does not reach the circulation
- Useful indicator of hepatic disease (especially biliary obstruction as it is mainly produced by the bile duct epithelium rather than as a result of hepatocellular damage)
- Relatively insensitive

LACTATE DEHYDROGENASE (LDH)

- Not liver specific
- Found in a number of other tissues, e.g. skeletal and cardiac muscle
- Elevated after restraint and haemolysis
- Not useful by itself in determination of hepatic disease

CREATINE KINASE (CK, CPK)

- Found mainly in skeletal muscle but also in cardiac and smooth muscle and brain
- Acts as a useful marker for muscle damage
  - Aids distinction between hepatic and muscle sources of AST and LDH
    - If CK is not elevated, increases in these enzymes strongly suggest hepatic disease
    - If CK is elevated, AST and LDH increases may be from liver or muscle, the latter due to physical exercise or tissue damage

AMMONIA

- Likely to reflect dietary protein and caecal microflora fermentation patterns rather than liver disease
- Assay difficult to perform in a practice situation (unless on-site laboratory facilities) as requires immediate analysis

BILE ACIDS

- Little information on bile acids in the rabbit
- Thought to be a sensitive indicator of liver function

- High levels indicate bile stasis
- Continual presence of food in the GIT and the practice of caecotrophy make dynamic testing pointless

CLEARANCE TESTING

- Cholephilic dye testing (sulfobromoph-thalein: BSP) and (indocyanine green: ICG) have been used to measure liver function in rabbits
- BSP is eliminated almost exclusively by the liver
- ICG is a sensitive test of liver function

KETONES AND BETA-HYDROXYBUTYRATE (BHB)

- Blood ketone levels may be increased with hepatic lipidosis
- Beta-hydroxybutyrate levels may measurably increase in DM and hepatic lipidosis

UREA

- Urea levels may be lowered in hepatic disease due to reduced production, especially in severe or chronic cases of insufficiency

BILIRUBIN

- Biliverdin rather than bilirubin is the major bile pigment in the rabbit, but bilirubin levels may be measurable
- Bilirubin levels reflect both hepatocellular damage and biliary tree function, but mainly the latter
- Laboratory rabbits have been reported with haemolytic anaemia associated with lymphosarcoma

Causes of an increase in bilirubin
- Bile duct obstruction
  - Hepatic coccidiosis
  - Hepatic neoplasia
  - Aflatoxicosis induced hepatic fibrosis
- VHD
- Haemolysis
- Large intestinal haemorrhage

BILIVERDIN

- No commercial test exists at present for this bile pigment

SERUM PROTEIN

- Hypoproteinaemia can occur in rabbits with significant long-term liver disease, due to decreased production
- Hypoalbuminaemia is often found in young rabbits affected by hepatic coccidiosis

COMMON LABORATORY ABNORMALITIES

SERUM PROTEIN ABNORMALITIES

TOTAL PROTEIN (TP)

- Total protein varies with breed and strain of rabbit
  - Polish > NZW > Dutch
- In NZW, TP is lower in immature animals and gradually increases with age

Causes of increased total protein

- Dehydration
- Hypovolaemia
- Prolonged hypothermia
- In late pregnancy, increased globulin may exceed decreased albumin
- Entire animals in breeding condition
- Chronic disease
- Immune mediated disease
- Heat stroke
- Shock
- Artefactual due to slow blood collection

Causes of decreased total protein

- Starvation
- Overhydration
- Protein losing nephropathies (glomeru-lonephropathy)
- Protein-losing enteropathies
- Advanced hepatic disease due to decreased production
- Pregnancy
- Adrenocortical stress or glucocorticoid administration
- Losses due to thermal burns, haemorrhage or flystrike

Albumin makes up approximately 60% of TP (higher than in most other mammals).

ALBUMIN

Causes of increased albumin

- Dehydration
  - Increased TP, albumin and globulin, A:G ratio normal
- Hypovolaemia

- May be higher in NZW females than males

Causes of decreased albumin

- Protein-losing nephropathies
- Protein-losing enteropathies
- Advanced hepatic disease due to decreased production
- Starvation/inappetance/reduced caecotrophy
- Pregnancy
- Old age
- Overhydration
- Excessive protein breakdown/loss
  - Sepsis
  - Severe trauma
  - Cachexia
  - Exudative losses: burns, flystrike

GLOBULIN

Causes of increased globulin

- Pregnancy (especially late pregnancy: alpha-globulins)
- Colostrum ingestion
- Acute infection
- Chronic disease
- Immune mediated disease
- Myeloproliferative disease
- Mycotic infection
- Coronaviral infection leads to dramatic increases (rare in pet rabbits – possibly non-existent without experimental inoculation)
- May be artefactually increased in lipaemic samples

FIBRINOGEN

- Limited correlation with inflammation in rabbits, but can be an indicator of cold stress
- Varies with age
  - Lower in young rabbits

SERUM PROTEIN ELECTROPHORESIS

Little work has been done on protein fractions in rabbits. Extrapolating from other species, one would expect the following:

Causes of increased alpha-globulins
- Acute tissue injury, inflammation, pyrexia
- Subacute inflammation, especially bacterial
- Glomerulonephritis and amyloidosis
- Internal abscessation (alpha-2 globulin)
- Late pregnancy

Causes of increased beta-globulins
- Acute tissue injury, inflammation, pyrexia (possibly fibrinogen rise also)
- Chronic inflammation (fibrinogen rise also)
- Glomerulonephritis and amyloidosis

Causes of increased gamma-globulins
- Subacute inflammation, especially bacterial
- Chronic inflammation
- Glomerulonephritis and amyloidosis
- Internal abscessation

URINALYSIS

COLLECTION METHOD

It is important to consider the collection method when evaluating results.

Soaked, discoloured bedding
This can be surprisingly useful, even if dried. Mix with water, shake, and test for haemoglobin using test strips.
- Dietary pigments in the urine are a common cause of reddish discoloration but do not react with haemoglobin test patches on dipsticks (e.g. Multistix, Bayer)

Free catch (or from clean litter tray)
- Liable to faecal and environmental contamination
- Useful at home for glucose sampling with reduced stress
- Observation of urination helpful
  - Midstream flow is predominantly from bladder
  - Early and especially late flow samples will also be affected in females by vaginal and cervical discharges
  - Uterine blood usually passed at end (active straining phase) of micturition

Bladder expression conscious, sedated or GA
- Reflex micturition often follows moderate pressure when palpating the bladder
- Manual expression possible, especially under sedation/GA
- Less contamination
- Does not differentiate urinary tract vs. genital tract

Catheterization
- Usually requires sedation/GA
- Less contamination than either method given above
- Does not differentiate urinary tract vs. genital tract in male
- Possible artefactual blood from catheterization trauma

Cystocentesis
- Risk of caecal puncture
- Possible contamination with intestinal fluid
- Possible artefactual blood from cystocentesis trauma

COMMON LABORATORY ABNORMALITIES

ANALYSIS METHOD

- Test dipsticks are only accurate for haemoglobin, pH, glucose and ketones
- Tests for leucocytes, nitrite, urobilinogen and relative density (SG) are inaccurate in rabbits
- Dipstick tests for protein are commonly positive and do not necessarily indicate renal disease
- Cytology is complicated by the normal presence of calcium crystals
  - Sampling the supernatant/sediment interface may be more rewarding, but cells may be distorted by centrifugation

TIME OF DAY

- Early morning samples are more concentrated, with higher cell, cast and bacteria yields
- Recently formed samples are less likely to have damage to cells or casts

PARAMETERS

Gross appearance
Normal
- Cloudy, due to suspended calcium crystals
- Varies from light yellow to red/brown due to dietary pigments

Clear
- Hypocalcaemia
- Renal failure
- Pregnancy
- Lactation
- Growing rabbit

Blood
- Always confirm apparent haematuria by test strip or microscopy
- Blood produced anywhere along urinary and genital tracts

- Differentiate source by observation and comparison of collection method
  - For example, in a mature intact doe, haematuria in a voided sample but no haematuria in a cystocentesis sample is strongly suggestive of uterine pathology.

Glucose
- Stress, e.g. of travelling to the surgery, or the stress of any underlying disease process
- Excessive, repeated presence of glucose in low stress surroundings is suggestive of altered energy metabolism
  - Undiscovered disease process
  - Hepatic lipidosis
  - Possibly DM
- Renal failure

Ketones
- Anorexia (even of only a few days duration)
- Hepatic lipidosis
- Pregnancy toxaemia
- DM

Sediment
Crystals
- Up to 50% of sample can be seen in normal rabbits
  - After centrifugation or settlement the crystals in the urine of the normal rabbit should resuspend when shaken
  - Those seen in 'sludge' remain as a solid mass
- Total absence may suggest
  - Hypocalcaemia
  - Renal failure
  - Pregnancy
  - Lactation
  - Growing rabbit

Cytology
White cells
- Small numbers not abnormal
- Urinary tract inflammation

- Genital tract inflammation (depending on sample source)

Red cells
- See Haematuria, p. 37

Casts
- Casts localize site to renal tubules

Neoplastic cells
Whilst lack of neoplastic cells does not rule out neoplasia, their presence can indicate both type and site of tumours.

Culture and sensitivity
- Bacterial culture and sensitivity performed on cystocentesed urine is the most reliable test for bacterial urinary tract infections
- Other methods of collection risk contamination

Relative density (specific gravity)
- Often difficult to measure because of the crystalline content of the urine

Increased relative density
- With azotaemia suggests pre-renal failure

Normal or decreased
- With azotaemia suggests primary renal failure

pH
- Normally 7–9; this does not indicate cystitis

- Aged samples may have falsely elevated pH
- Decreased pH
  - Fasting
  - Fever
  - Pregnancy toxaemia
  - Hepatic lipidosis

Proteinuria
- Traces in adults usually of no clinical significance
- Small amounts of albumin may be seen in normal young rabbits
- Very dilute (< 1.020) urine with protein present is more significant
- Amyloidosis is clinically rare
- Renal failure
  - Proteinuria seen from very early on in the disease process
  - One of the earliest indicators of renal damage
  - Seen before raised blood urea/creatinine
  - Post-renal proteinuria seen with inflammation of lower urinary tract
- Urine protein/urine creatinine ratios
  - Raised values may indicate glomerular disease
  - < 0.6 suggested as normal

Encephalitozoon spore evaluation
- Gram or trichrome stains can reveal *Encephalitozoon cuniculi*
- PCR techniques are being investigated

FAECAL ANALYSIS

Distinguish between true faeces and caecotrophs
- Many cases presented as having diarrhoea and 'clagging' are really presenting with normal caecotrophs which have not been consumed (see Caecotroph accumulation, p. 13)

NORMAL APPEARANCE

True faeces (hard faeces)
- Dry, hard pellets 3–10 mm in diameter
- Need prolonged soaking or maceration to allow microscopy
- Composed almost entirely of pieces of undigested plant remains > 0.5 mm in length

- The presence of large numbers of yeasts (*Cyniclomyces* sp.) is normal

Caecotrophs
- Normally soft (a thick paste consistency) and surrounded by thin coat of mucus
- Not normally observed by the owner
  - Should be ingested directly from the anus by the rabbit
- Consider physical and pathological reasons for the observable presence of caecotrophs
- Consist predominantly of microbes and digested particulate matter
  - Little or no undigested plant remains > 0.5 mm in length
  - Presence of larger pieces of undigested plant remains suggest an alteration in GI motility

Common organisms found on wet preparation or Gram-stained cytology of normal caecotrophs include:
- Gram negative bacilli
- Bacteroides
- Large metachromic bacilli
- Many other bacteria
- Various motile protozoa
- Large numbers of *Cyniclomyces* sp. yeasts

PRESENCE OF PARASITES

Ova or oocysts of various nematodes and coccidia can be found simply on examination of a faecal wet preparation smear, but standard flotation techniques can be used to improve recovery of the organisms and also to provide quantitative analysis.

Passalurus ambiguus and *P. nonannulatus*
- Typical 'pinworm' ova
- Ovoid but asymmetrically flattened with a cap at one end

- Common (?normal) and usually apathogenic inhabitant of the GIT
  - May even have beneficial properties

Other nematodes
- Various trichostrongylid worms (e.g. *Graphidium strigosum* [Europe] and *Obeliscoides cuniculi* [USA])
  - Larger and more regular ovoid eggs
  - Very occasionally seen in pet rabbits
    — More common in wild rabbits
  - Should be considered abnormal

Coccidia
See Coccidiosis, p. 179.
- A number of *Eimeria* species exist
- Vary tremendously in their pathogenicity
- Several are completely apathogenic
- Particularly common in young rabbits
- Some species can cause severe diarrhoea or liver damage
- Combination of oocyst morphology and measurement is used to determine which species of coccidia are present, to better predict the likely significance of coccidia in a faecal sample

Cryptosporidium
- Occasional parasite of rabbits
- Special stains (acid-fast, immunofluorescence) necessary
- ELISA tests may be available

Bacteriology
- Infectious bacterial enteritis is rare in individual pet rabbits
- *Escherichia coli*, *Campylobacter* and *Salmonella* can cause outbreaks of disease in colonies
  - Particularly in kits prior to weaning
  - None of these organisms is found in normal rabbit faeces
    — *E. coli* can be present as an opportunist when other GI pathology, such as reduced motility, is present

- *Clostridium spiroforme*
  - Responsible for enterotoxaemia
  - Occasionally can be seen as large Gram positive semicircular or spiral shaped bacteria in faecal smears
  - Anaerobic culture of the organism is required to confirm its identity
- *Clostridium piliforme*
  - Causes Tyzzer's disease
  - Cannot be detected on routine faecal examination
  - PCR tests are available in some countries

PRESENCE OF MUCUS

- A coat of mucus is a normal finding around caecotrophs
- Mucus passed with hard faeces or mucus passed on its own is usually evidence of a disruption of the normal GI motility pattern rather than evidence of colitis
- Clear, gelatinous mucus passed without any faecal material is a characteristic sign of true mucoid enteropathy syndrome
  - Dysautonomia which causes a complete cessation in colonic motility, whilst the colon continues to secrete mucus which eventually may overflow through sheer volume from the anus

CEREBROSPINAL FLUID (CSF) ANALYSIS

INDICATIONS

- Further investigation of suspected inflammatory, infectious or neoplastic lesions of the CNS
- Widely used in laboratory situations as a model for investigation of meningitis and drug penetration into CSF
  - Catheter implantation techniques allow later repeated samples to be taken from conscious rabbits

TECHNIQUE

Cisterna magna
The cisterna magna is sampled via an atlanto-occipital approach. The rabbit is anaesthetized and placed in lateral recumbency. The neck is clipped and prepared for surgery. The nose is pointed down tight to the chest, but avoiding airway compromise. A 40 mm × 0.65 mm spinal needle (23g 1.5") is introduced horizontally in the midline just caudal to the occipital ridge. The needle is advanced towards the nose until the dura and subarachnoid membranes are 'popped'. The stylet can be removed and the sample should be allowed to drip out naturally from the needle rather than being aspirated.

Lumbosacral tap
Lumbosacral tap is described as being similar to the procedure in a dog. The epidural space of a rabbit is 0.75–2.5 cm beneath the skin surface.

CSF ANALYSIS

Normal values are listed below; however, there are no readily available guidelines on how to interpret values differing from these values in the rabbit.

CSF constituents of normal rabbits
- WBC: 1–7 cells/mm^3
- Lymphocytes: 40–79%
- Monocytes: 21–60%
- Glucose: 4.16 mmol/l
- Urea nitrogen: 14.28 mmol/l

- Creatinine: 1500 μmol/l
- Cholesterol: 0.825 mmol/l
- Total protein: 59 g/l
- Alkaline phosphatase: 50 iu/l
- Sodium: 149 mmol/l
- Potassium: 3 mmol/l
- Chloride: 127 mmol/l

- Calcium: 1.35 mmol/l
- Magnesium: 0.9 mmol/l
- Phosphate: 0.75 mmol/l

Additionally bacterial culture and sensitivity or PCR techniques can be used in cases where infectious organisms are suspected.

SECTION 3
ORGAN SYSTEMS

CARDIOVASCULAR DISEASE

With the exception of atherosclerosis (for which the rabbit has been used as a model of human disease), there is relatively little information available regarding cardiac disease in the rabbit. With recent advances in healthcare, rabbits can be expected to live longer and often with a greater degree of freedom to exercise than with the traditional hutch bound animal, and it is likely that cardiac disease will become a more commonly recognized problem in the rabbit.

ATHEROSCLEROSIS AND ARTERIAL MINERALIZATION

Arteriosclerosis is defined as any condition characterized by thickening and loss of elasticity of the arterial walls. *Atherosclerosis* is a form of arteriosclerosis characterized by deposition of yellowish plaques of cholesterol and other lipid materials within the intima of large and medium-sized arteries.

Atherosclerosis

- Develops as a consequence of hyper-cholesterolaemia
- Some laboratory strains of rabbit (Watanebe) have been bred to develop hypercholesterolaemia
- In most rabbits, hypercholesterolaemia is a consequence of excessive fat intake
- Other concurrent signs of hypercholesterolaemia may be seen, e.g. cholesterol deposits within the cornea
- Atherosclerosis lesions (atheromas) form within the major arteries, particularly the aorta
- Potentially lead to cardiac failure through restriction of cardiac output and consequent effects on bloodflow and pressure dynamics. Weight loss is a common reported presentation
- More likely to cause embolic disease as portions of atheroma detach and enter the bloodstream
  - Seizures
  - Vestibular disease
  - Acute cardiac failure

Arteriosclerosis

- Mineralization of the aortic arch
- Often associated with mineralization of kidney tissues
- Clinical signs of renal disease with impaired calcium excretion
- Exact pathogenesis of the hypercalcaemia has not been determined
- Mineralization of the kidneys and of the aorta may be seen on radiographs, sometimes as an incidental finding

CARDIOMYOPATHY

There are a number of possible causes of cardiomyopathy (myocardial fibrosis) in rabbits, although a number of these have only been shown to cause it experimentally.

- Dietary
  - Vitamin E deficiency
- Bacterial infections
  - *Salmonella*
  - *Pasteurella*
  - Tyzzer's disease
- Viral infections
  - Experimental administration of coronavirus
- Parasitic infections
  - Encephalitozoonosis
- Stress
  - Overcrowding
- Exogenous catecholamines
  - Hypoxaemia and coronary vasoconstriction
- Ketamine/xylazine anaesthesia
  - Theorized to be a catecholamine-like effect of the adrenoceptor agonist

ORGAN SYSTEMS

- Idiopathic/breed related
  - Giant breeds are particularly susceptible

INVESTIGATION OF SUSPECTED CARDIAC DISEASE

Presentation
- Clinically healthy
  - Murmur or dysrhythmia noted during routine examination or during anaesthetic monitoring
- Evidence of congenital cardiac disease
  - Failure to thrive, failure to gain weight
  - Collapse
- Evidence of decompensated cardiac disease
  - Weakness, lethargy
  - Weight loss
  - Dyspnoea
  - Collapse
  - Abdominal distension
- Concurrent disease which is affecting cardiac function

Classification
Murmurs
- Intensity graded I–VI
- Point of maximum intensity and radiation
- Timing and duration, pitch, gallop beats, etc., are usually very difficult to determine because of the normally very rapid heart rate (130–325 beats per minute), especially in small breeds

Dysrhythmias
Unless severe, dysrhythmias are difficult to characterize or even appreciate on auscultation – electrocardiography is usually necessary.

KEY HISTORY

- Age and breed
  - Cardiomyopathy seen especially in giant rabbits
  - Some laboratory rabbit breeds are specifically susceptible to atherosclerosis, e.g. Watanebe – hypercholesterolaemia even on extreme low fat diets
  - Congenital defects such as ventricular septum defects can affect rabbit kits, but rabbit kits with apparently innocent murmurs also occur
- Diet
  - Vitamin E deficiency can cause cardiomyopathy
  - High fat diets can induce atherosclerosis
  - Excessive calcium and vitamin D_3 supplementation may be a cause of aortic mineralization
- Access to potential toxins
  - Foxglove (cardiac glycosides)
  - Deadly nightshade (atropine; but most rabbits are resistant due to circulating atropinesterase)
  - Others
- Previous disease history
  - Rabbits surviving *Salmonella*, *Pasteurella* and Tyzzer's disease infections can have cardiomyopathy
  - Encephalitozoonosis can be a cause of cardiomyopathy and possibly of dysrhythmia
  - Renal disease can result in hypercalcaemia with consequent aortic mineralization
- Anaesthetic history
  - Excessive stimulation by adrenaline and alpha$_2$-adrenoceptor agonists have been suggested as possible causes of cardiomyopathy

Physical examination
- Where possible, characterization of murmur and rhythm

- Mucosal colour
  - Difficult to assess in many breeds
  - Iris colour in albino breeds
  - Vulva/prepuce
  - Pulse oximetry
- Assessment of peripheral circulation
  - Warmth of feet and ear tips
  - Capillary refill time
  - Pulse quality
  - Blood pressure measurement
- Respiratory rate +/– dyspnoea
- Ascites or ventral/peripheral oedema
- Exophthalmos
- Signs of other disease processes

Decision-making

- Is this an incidental finding? Is it congenital?
- Is this secondary to some other disease process?
  - Anaemia, pyrexia, toxaemia, ketosis
- Are there clinical signs of cardiac disease?

Diagnostic approach

- Electrocardiography
  - Normal heart rate varies from 130 to 325 beats/minute
  - Normal respiratory rate is between 30 and 60 breaths/minute
  - Respiratory rate is sinus with **no** sinus arrhythmia
- Echocardiography
  - In the rabbit the 'tricuspid' valve only has two cusps
  - The pulmonary artery is markedly muscular compared to felines
- Haematology and biochemistry
  - To rule out systemic disease, assess renal function, look for signs of inflammatory disease

- Thoracic radiography
  - But will require GA, which could exacerbate clinical cardiac disease

MANAGEMENT OF DECOMPENSATED CARDIAC DISEASE

- Clinical problems
  - Pulmonary oedema
  - Pleural effusion
  - Hepatomegaly
- Management – diuretics
  - Frusemide
    - Variable response of rabbit nephrons to loop diuretics
    - 1–4 mg/kg IV/IM q4–12 h
    - Longer term 1–2 mg/kg PO q8–24 h
  - Other diuretics
    - Bendrofluadride has been suggested in cases where calcium-salt-related urinary tract disease is a concurrent issue
  - 'Natural diuretics'
    - Yarrow, dandelion
  - Vasodilators
    - Nitroglycerin ointment 2%, 3 mm transdermally q6–12 h
- ACEIs
  - Enalapril maleate 0.25–0.5 mg/kg PO q24–48 h
- Digoxin
  - For cases of valvular regurgitation or dilated cardiomyopathy
  - 0.005–0.01 mg/kg q24–48 h
- Rest?
  - Although strict cage rest is indicated in canine and feline patients, physical activity is an important component of gut motility in the rabbit

ORGAN SYSTEMS

RESPIRATORY DISEASES

GENERAL APPROACH TO RESPIRATORY DISEASE

- Respiratory distress is a common presentation in rabbits, but differentiation of the various causes can be difficult
- Observe the rate, pattern and character of the rabbit's respiration whilst in an unstressed rested state
  - In the travelling container before handling
  - Loose on the floor of the consulting room while a history is being taken
  - Encourage owners to bring in video evidence of the respiratory signs that have been noted, especially if episodic
  - Be aware that the rabbit is an obligate nasal breather – unless in extreme respiratory distress, rabbits do not pant or mouth breathe; mouth breathing is a very poor prognostic sign
- After this initial observation, it may be appropriate to consider stabilization (oxygen tent, cage rest to overcome travelling stress, benzodiazepines if particularly stressed) before proceeding to further examination
- Perform a full clinical examination, paying particular attention to:
  - Skin lesions or asymmetry of the nasal area
  - Discharges (unilateral or bilateral) from the nose (or matted hair on the inner carpi)
  - Airflow present at both nares? Respiratory signs worsened when either naris is blocked?
  - Palpation of the skull, larynx and neck area
    - Rabbits do not often display a 'cough on tracheal palpation' response, even in the presence of overt tracheobronchial disease

- Oral examination using an otoscope, and if necessary completed under sedation/GA
- Palpate the thorax for thoracic wall masses or trauma, position of apex beat: compressibility is difficult to assess as it varies dramatically between breeds
- Auscultate the nasal chamber, laryngeal region and entire thorax to evaluate extent of lungfields and assess normality of cardiac and respiratory sounds
  - Because of the obligate nasal airway, upper respiratory noise is frequently heard when auscultating the chest and is easily misinterpreted
- Percuss the thorax for evidence of increased or decreased resonance

AIRWAY DISORDERS

Nares
Myxomatosis
- Oedema of the lips, nares and facial skin occurs in myxomatosis
- Diagnosis is based on the almost pathognomonic clinical appearance, with definitive diagnosis on electron microscopy
- There is no specific cure for myxomatosis, although supportive care and good nursing may enable recovery in some mildly affected rabbits (see Myxomatosis, p. 188)

Rabbit syphilis
- *Treponema cuniculi* affects the mucocutaneous junctions of the face
- The genitals are also often affected, as with myxomatosis, but there is not generally oedema, and it is usually possible to differentiate the two diseases just on physical appearance

- Dark field microscopy or silver stains identify the organism
- *T. cuniculi* is sensitive to a number of antibiotics
- (See Treponemiasis, p. 193)

Trauma to the nasal area/lips
- Physical, chemical or thermal
- There is often a history of fighting, damaged jagged water drinkers or wire, or access to caustic chemicals
- Treatment generally involves providing supportive care, including analgesia to minimize the risk of anorexia
- Supportive fluids and supplementary feeding may be necessary if the rabbit is struggling to eat

Nasal chamber (rhinitis)
Inhaled irritants
- Ammonia
  - Poor hutch hygiene
- Dust
  - Poor quality hay, straw, sawdust bedding
- Various household/DIY products
  - Shed/garage housed rabbits
    — petroleum products
    — creosote
    — paints
  - Indoor housed rabbits
    — air fresheners
    — disinfectants
    — perfumes
    — talcum powder

Foreign bodies
- Particularly ends of pieces of hay which enter either nostril during feeding
  - Rabbits cannot visualize objects directly in front of the nose

Infections
- Local
  - Rhinitis associated with *Pasteurella, Bordetella, Staphylococcus*

  - Mucocutaneous dermatosis associated with *Treponema paraluis-cuniculi* infection
- Systemic
  - Pasteurellosis
  - Myxomatosis

Sinuses
- Rabbits do not have a frontal sinus
- There are conchal and maxillary sinuses and occasionally these are involved in infectious (bacterial) rhinitis

Nasopharynx
- Caudal nasal foreign bodies
- Eustachian foreign bodies
  - Because of the poor cough response and lack of vomition in rabbits, caudal nasal FBs are less common than rostral nasal FBs and have usually passed back from the nostril rather than forward from the pharynx
  - The most common FBs are hay, grass seeds and shafts of hair
  - In occasional cases the FB is found to have penetrated the Eustachian tube
  - Most FBs require rhinoscopy (endoscopic examination with a 1.2–2.7 mm diameter semi-rigid or rigid endoscope with or without irrigation/biopsy sheath) to identify and remove the offending structure
- Pharyngeal abscessation
  - Abscesses in the caudal oral cavity or pharyngeal region are a common consequence of dental disease and occasionally these impinge on the airway, restricting free airflow

Larynx/trachea
- Laryngeal granuloma
- Foreign body
  - Iatrogenic aspiration of dental equipment (burr) or debris during dentistry

Approach

- GA examination, teeth and larynx
- Endoscopic examination
  - Nasal cavity, nasopharynx, larynx, trachea, pleural space
  - Including taking samples for cytology, bacteriology or histopathology
- Radiography. (This presents problems. Conscious dorsoventral radiography may be possible, and may assist in assessing some differentials, such as unilateral pleural disease, abscessation, thymoma or advanced metastatic neoplasia, but rarely provides a fully diagnostic radiograph. The decision to proceed with general anaesthesia to enable inflated dorsoventral and lateral views, together with further diagnostic tests such as endoscopic examinations or bronchoalveolar lavage must be made on an individual case basis; often empirical symptomatic treatment in an attempt to stabilize the case will have to take precedence.)
- CT/MRI (to demonstrate permanent remodelling of turbinate structures)
- Bronchoalveolar lavage
  - Cytology
  - Bacteriology

Therapeutics

- Address underlying husbandry factors
- Primary resolution where possible (removal of FB; surgery for abscess, granuloma, etc.)
- Antibiosis +/– supportive therapy (oxygen, humidification of air, analgesics/anti-inflammatories)
- Nebulization
  - Various antibiotics and other materials can be 'nebulized', i.e. made into a mist which the rabbit breathes in, with the effect of humidifying the respiratory surfaces and delivering therapeutic substances directly to the necessary site

PULMONARY DISORDERS

Alveolar diseases
Haemorrhage

- Less common in rabbits than in dogs and cats because of the lack of opportunity for road traffic accidents and similar traumatic incidents
- Coagulopathies are rare, with the exception of disseminated intravascular coagulopathy as a consequence of caliciviral hepatopathy
- Haemorrhage from airway or pulmonary neoplasia, abscesses or granulomata

Oedema

- Raised capillary pressure or increased capillary permeability
  - Cardiac failure
  - Paraquat or inhalant toxins
  - Heat stroke, electric shock
  - Drowning
  - ?Allergic
  - Secondary to other disorders, e.g. pneumonia, hypoproteinaemia
  - Excessive use of parenteral fluid therapy

Exudation

- Bronchopneumonia
  - Lower airway infections, e.g. *Pasteurella*, *Bordetella*
  - Inhaled irritants, e.g. smoke, ammonia
  - Aspirated food material
    - Rare, because of the lack of vomition
    - Seen occasionally following difficult force feeding
    - Seen as a terminal consequence of mucoid enteropathy syndrome
- Neoplasia (primary or secondary)
- Localized abscessation

May cause bronchial obstruction, lung lobe collapse, secondary pneumonia, pleural effusion.

Granulomatous disease
- Rare
  - Mycobacteria
  - Fungi
  - Foreign body response to a grass awn or piece of straw

Signs
- Dyspnoea/tachypnoea
  - Coughing is unusual
  - What owners perceive to be cough is more likely to be sneeze or 'snuffle' response to upper respiratory tract infection
- Exercise intolerance
  - Depending on husbandry system this may not be observed by the owner
- Debility
  - Weakness
  - Weight loss
  - Inappetance
  - GI disturbances, e.g. inability to ingest caecotrophs due to worsening of respiratory problem when trying to bend to reach the anus
- Signs of concurrent upper respiratory tract, ocular or systemic infection in pasteurellosis

Findings
- Cyanosis and mucous membrane pallour are difficult to detect until severe because of the difficulty observing the gums and because of the natural variation in oral membrane colour. May be more obvious in the iris coloration of 'red-eyed' breeds

Auscultation
- Can be difficult in some rabbits because of noise from the upper respiratory tract
- Rales, vesicular sounds and rhonchi may be present
- Heart sounds may be muffled or absent in the presence of consolidation or masses (neoplasia, abscessation)

Investigations
- Haematology
  - Leucocytosis or neutrophilia in bronchopneumonia
  - Anaemia may suggest haemorrhage but is common with any chronic disease
- Radiography
  - Difficult due to difficulty restraining manually, rapid respiratory rate and risks of GA in a rabbit with respiratory compromise
  - Where possible, radiography is the investigative method of choice
- Bronchoalveolar lavage
  - Useful for obtaining cytological specimens to differentiate inflammatory causes
  - May be possible in hypnotized (tranced) rabbits, but more usually requires GA
- Endoscopy
  - Again requires GA
  - Evaluation both via the trachea (allowing direct sampling of any discharges for cytology and bacteriology) and also via thoracotomy allowing examination of the pleural surface of the lungs and fine needle aspiration or biopsy of any lesions for evaluation by cytology, histopathology and bacteriology

Interstitial diseases
- Rare in rabbits
- Metastatic neoplasms
  - Particularly mammary and uterine carcinomas
- Paraquat poisoning

Signs, findings and investigation
- Similar to those of alveolar diseases
- Likely to require lung biopsy (possibly via endoscopy) to reach a specific diagnosis
- Prognosis in all cases is poor

Miscellaneous diseases
- Lung lobe torsion
- Lung lobe rupture

ORGAN SYSTEMS

- Lung lobe collapse (usually due to compression of the lung, or occlusion of a major bronchus) by pulmonary, pleural or mediastinal masses or fluid accumulation

Signs, findings and investigation
- Similar to those of alveolar diseases

Management of pulmonary disorders
General therapy
- Maintain an open airway
- Maintain warmth
- Encourage moderately restricted exercise
  - Complete rest is contraindicated because of the necessity to maintain GI motility
- Ensure adequate hydration
- Provide parenteral fluid therapy if necessary
- Provide oxygen therapy in an emergency

Specific therapy
- Surgical resection
  - Lung lobe torsion
  - Discrete abscesses
  - Granulomas
  - Neoplasms
  - (Is rarely possible)
- Diuresis in cases of oedema
- Antibiotic therapy for bronchopneumonia and for inoperable abscessation
  - Initially aimed at *Pasteurella* and *Bordetella*
    - Fluoroquinolones
    - Tetracyclines
  - Where possible adjusted according to bacteriology results
  - Nebulized antibiosis should be considered in addition to systemic treatment
- Use of mucolytics (bromhexine, acetylcysteine) may help clearance of exudates and may improve antibiotic penetration

Metastatic neoplasia carries a poor prognosis. Advice of an oncologist should be sought regarding potential chemotherapeutics, but the response at this stage is generally poor.

PLEURAL AND MEDIASTINAL DISEASES

Effusions
Usually limited to one side of the chest where localized lesions responsible
- Blood
  - Traumatic, e.g. bite wound, fractured rib
  - From a mass, e.g. neoplasm, lung abscess
  - Coagulopathy, e.g. due to terminal VHD, warfarin poisoning
- Pus (pleurisy)
  - Penetrating wounds of thoracic wall or oesophagus
    - *Staphylococcus* if simple penetration
    - Anaerobes if bite wounds
  - Rupture of a pneumonic or mediastinal abscess
  - Foreign body, e.g. grass seed
  - Extension of pneumonia
    - Usually via abscess (see above)
- Chyle
  - Rupture of the lymphatic system as a consequence of trauma, neoplasia or unknown factors
- Modified transudate
  - Congestive heart failure or obstruction to venous return
  - Lung lobe torsion
  - Ruptured diaphragm
  - Fluid leakage associated with a neoplasm
- True transudate
  - Hypoproteinaemia
- Air (pneumothorax or pneumediastinum)
  - Traumatic
  - Associated with foreign body, abscess or tumour

Signs
- Tachypnoea and dyspnoea, especially when stressed
- Weight loss in chronic cases
- Ascites in cardiac failure and hypoproteinaemia

Findings
- Signs of anaemia
  - Pale mucous membranes
  - Weak pulse
- Cyanosis
  - Difficult to assess except in albino breeds, where the iris is a useful indicator
- Auscultation and percussion
  - Particularly useful in unilateral cases where reduction in cardiac and respiratory sounds and altered resonance are noted on the affected side
  - Less obvious in bilateral cases
- Subcutaneous oedema or ascites in cardiac failure and hypoproteinaemia

Investigations
- Radiography. (Depending on the degree of compromise of the animal's respiration and temperament of the animal a conscious dorsoventral radiograph may be indicated before considering chemical restraint; inverting the animal for a ventrodorsal view should be avoided.)
- Thoracocentesis (+/– abdominocentesis) with appropriate testing of any aspirated fluid (cytology, specific gravity, protein)
- Haematology and biochemistry

Space-occupying lesions
- Thymoma/thymic lymphosarcoma
  - *Note*: In the rabbit the normal thymus remains large throughout adult life, and there is normally little or no radiographically evident cranial lungfield
- Pulmonary or mediastinal abscess
- Abscess of the body wall
- Cardiomegaly
- Neoplasia

(Due to the anatomic arrangement of abdominal structures, and also the size differential between abdominal and thoracic contents, herniation of abdominal content into the thoracic cavity is likely to be fatal when it occurs.)

Signs
Only become evident when a significant portion of thoracic volume is occupied.
- Dyspnoea (due to reduction in ventilation as with pleural fluid, or due to pressure on major airways)
- Dysphagia or regurgitation due to pressure on the oesophagus
- Exophthalmos as a consequence of increased pressure on the jugular vein (especially thymoma)

Findings
- Often very little to find other than the presenting clinical signs
- Occasionally muffling or displacement of heart or respiratory sounds may be noticed on auscultation

Investigations
- As for pleural effusions:
  - Radiography (with care)
  - Thoracocentesis if fluid present
  - Haematology and biochemistry
  - Ultrasonography
  - Fine needle aspirate for cytology (+/– bacteriology) where the mass can be accessed. (*Note*: Due to the strong possibility of a mass being an abscess, and proximity of major blood vessels in many cases, 'Trucut' biopsies are usually contraindicated.)

Treatment of pleural and mediastinal disorders
Stabilization/palliation
- Repeated drainage of pleural fluid/air to restore normal ventilation
- Oxygen therapy

ORGAN SYSTEMS

Specific therapy
Pyothorax (pleurisy)
- Placement of an indwelling catheter or chest drain to allow repeated drainage
- Systemic antibacterial therapy
  - Where possible take samples for bacteriological examination before initiating antibiosis
  - Aim initially for broad spectrum cover, particularly against *Pasteurella*, *Staphylococcus* and anaerobes
    — Fluoroquinolone and metronidazole
    — Tetracyclines and metronidazole
    — Cephalexin
  - Change therapy as appropriate once results of bacteriological examination are known
- Local therapy
  - Lavage of the pleural space using sterile saline +/− hyaluronidase in an attempt to remove inspissated purulent debris

- Instillation of antibacterials into the pleural space
  — Fluoroquinolones
  — Metronidazole
  — Soluble cephalosporins

Cardiac effusion
(See Cardiovascular disease, p. 91.)

Pneumothorax
- Often self-resolving with simple palliative management
- Use of a valved or negative pressure chest drain may be indicated

Solid masses
- Surgical resection of thymic neoplasms has been reported
- Other neoplasms and abscesses are unlikely to be resectable unless involving the extremity of the caudal lung lobes
- Abscesses may decrease in size or at least be controlled by intensive systemic antibiosis

NEUROMUSCULAR SYSTEM AND DISORDERS

GENERAL APPROACH TO A NEUROLOGICAL CASE

Neurological symptoms, particularly 'head tilt', are a common reason for presentation of a rabbit to the veterinary surgeon.

Approach to the case
- Full history, including:
  - Possibility of trauma
  - Access to toxins or unaccustomed foodstuffs
  - Recent medications
  - Proximity of other rabbits
- General clinical examination, including:
  - Assessment of mentation (when not stressed)
  - Head position
  - Ability to stand, abnormalities of gait
    — Encourage owners to bring in video footage of the abnormality if episodic
  - Ocular examination for strabismus and spontaneous or positional nystagmus

Investigation of neurological disease can be frustrating, since rabbits have a highly flexed plantigrade stance at rest, and tend to 'freeze' when stressed, and give inconsistent responses to some neurologic tests purely as an innate lack of responsiveness. There is also a risk of causing spinal dislocation or fracture when attempting some of the tests, such as hemiwalking or wheelbarrow tests, which would be performed on dogs and cats. However, with these limitations, the same battery of tests as performed on canine or feline patients can be considered.

Key objectives in investigation of neurological disease

- Are the presenting signs caused by a neurological disease, or by some other illness?
- If neurological, what is the duration of the signs; are they acute or gradual in onset?
- Is the lesion intracranial, spinal or elsewhere?
- Is the lesion unifocal or multifocal?
- What is the location of the lesion?
- Can a definitive diagnosis, or prognosis, be arrived at, with or without appropriate diagnostic tests?

CAUSES OF NEUROLOGICAL AND NEUROMUSCULAR DISEASE

Encephalitozoon cuniculi

- Intracellular microsporidian parasite
  - Can infect a wide range of mammalian and some avian hosts
  - Has become important in recent decades as a zoonotic disease of human immunocompromised patients
  - Has also been implicated as a disease-causing agent on fox fur farms and as one cause of 'fading puppy syndrome'
- Spread between rabbits via the urine
  - Infectious spores are either ingested or inhaled
  - Trans-placental transmission was experimentally found to be possible during the acute phase of infection, but is uncommon
- In rabbits *E. cuniculi* primarily affects two tissues:
  - Renal parenchyma
  - Central nervous system

- In the acute stage of infection, heart, lung and liver may also be affected
- In renal parenchyma, the organism causes foci of granulomatous inflammation which eventually scar over leaving pinhead white pitted areas on the kidney surface at post-mortem examination. The renal stage of infection is usually asymptomatic, but severe infections potentially could contribute to renal insufficiency
- In the CNS, the organism encysts, and clinically important lesions (such as suppurative granulomatous meningoencephalitis, astrogliosis and perivascular lymphocytic infiltration) do not occur until at least 1 month after experimental inoculation
  - It has been suggested that it is rupture of the cysts rather than the infection itself that causes the marked pathological changes that lead to clinical disease
  - Numbers of cysts involved and trigger factors which initiate cyst rupture have not been investigated
  - Neurological manifestations in rabbits infected by the parasite have been described since as early as 1922
- Clinical signs vary with the site within the CNS that is affected and include 'head tilt', posterior paresis, urinary incontinence, and vague signs such as a stiff rear gait, tremors and altered behaviour
  - In pet rabbits encephalitozoonosis appears to be by far the most common cause of 'head tilt'
- Serological testing is available
  - Many laboratories simply report the result as positive or negative rather than producing an accurate titre
  - Until recently, the only need for testing of rabbits was as a screening test before introducing new stock into a laboratory colony
  - Some laboratories are now reporting results in terms of titres

ORGAN SYSTEMS

○ Positive serology is at present not a confirmation that *E. cuniculi* is the cause of the disease process, and seroconversion rates within the 'normal' pet rabbit population are at present unknown, but thought to be around 50%

○ Since clinical disease rarely occurs less than 1 month post infection, a negative serological titre probably rules out *E. cuniculi* as the causative agent

• Definitive diagnosis is by the histological demonstration of granulomatous inflammation associated with the Gram-positive, carbol–fuchsin positive organisms in the CNS at post mortem

○ The situation is still not clear since, in some cases, granulomatous foci occur without obvious association with *E. cuniculi* organisms

• Fenbendazole has been shown *in vivo* to be effective, not against clinical disease, but in elimination of the organism from naturally infected rabbits and in prevention of infection and serological conversion in experimentally inoculated animals

○ Treatment duration, and ancilliary treatments must take into account the presence and infectivity of the parasite in contaminated bedding and environment

○ Dry spores at 22°C can remain infective for over a month, whilst moist spores can remain infective for 98 days

Vestibular disease

• Peripheral vestibular disease is generally due to otitis interna, most commonly as an extension of a chronic otitis media

○ The most common organisms involved are *Pasteurella multocida* and *Bordetella bronchiseptica* from the upper respiratory tract

○ Also *Escherischia coli*, *Proteus mirabilis*, *Staphylococcus aureus*, *Pseudomonas aeruginosa*

○ Ear mites *Psoroptes cuniculi* from an otitis externa

• Central vestibular or cerebellar disease can again be caused by any of the above bacterial pathogens, but also by *Toxoplasma gondi* and *Encephalitozoon cuniculi*, and presumably *Neospora caninum*

○ In the USA, *Baylisascaris procyonis*, a racoon nematode is a common cause in rabbits with outdoor access

○ Other canid or felid tapeworms potentially could cause similar migrations

• Other possible causes include:
○ Neoplasia
○ Cerebrovascular accidents
○ Emboli
— Cerebrovascular accidents and emboli have no specific treatments, and are difficult to diagnose without MRI or CAT scanning

• Cerebral mycoses (unlikely in the UK)
• Toxicoses
○ Lead and some plant toxins

Intracranial neoplasia
Medullary and pituitary teratomas and pituitary adenomas have been reported.

Baylisascaris procyonis

• Visceral larval migrans is a serious problem in certain parts of the USA

○ The racoon (*Procyon lotor*) is a wild animal which, similar to foxes in the UK, has found a niche scavenging from human dustbins

○ *Baylisascaris procyonis* is a common intestinal nematode of the racoon, and eggs are shed in large numbers in its faeces

○ These contaminate the ground and can be ingested by rabbits allowed outdoor grazing access, even in enclosed gardens

— Contamination of hay and straw food or bedding materials has also been implicated

○ The ova remain infective in the environment for many months

○ Once ingested by a rabbit, the larvae migrate around the rabbit's body, and in particular can invade the brain where even small larval numbers can cause head tilt, circling, ataxia, opisthotonos and tremors

○ Treatment is not possible

○ Aberrant migration of *Ascaris columnaris* (a parasite of the skunk, stoat, weasel and Siberian polecat) has also been reported in Europe

Listeriosis

• Listeriosis has been reported from rabbits
  ○ Seems less common than in ruminants
• Meningoencephalitis associated with *Listeria monocytogenes* has been reported to cause severe torticollis
  ○ Tetracyclines should be effective in early stages if ante-mortem or colony diagnosis can be made
  ○ Reproductive disease in females (metritis, abortions) has also been reported

Traumatic spinal disease

• Trauma to the lumbar spine at L6 or L7 is the most common reason for loss of neurological function to the hindlimbs
• The injury can occur due to improper handling, but also occurs when caged rabbits (which may be osteopaenic due to a combination of dietary factors and inadequate exercise) are startled and jump or 'thump' hard
  ○ The heavy hindlimbs twist around the lumbosacral junction
  ○ Luxation of the intervertebral joints and intervertebral discs is also possible
• Assessment of the case is much the same as for spinal lesions in canine and feline patients
  ○ Testing of movement, proprioception, reflexes, skin sensation, bladder and

perineal tone, and deep pain sensation, give an impression of the degree of compromise of the spinal cord

○ Radiography confirms the diagnosis; mild cases may respond to conservative support +/– anti-inflammatory therapy

○ More aggressive management (spinal decompression, spinal fracture fixation) are not widely reported, but could well be considered in rare cases

Muscular weakness

• A syndrome known as 'floppy rabbit syndrome' is one of the more frequent neurological presentations in pet rabbits
  ○ Animals present with an acute onset of generalized weakness and minimal response to external stimuli
  ○ There are many possible causes, and potential medical causes of collapse or apathy need to be thoroughly investigated
  ○ However, in some cases there appears to be no obvious underlying medical condition
• Proposed aetiologies/differentials in these cases include:
  ○ 'Lettuce poisoning'
  ○ Hypomagnesaemia
  ○ Hypokalaemia
  ○ Hypercalcaemia
  ○ Encephalitozoonosis
  ○ Toxoplasmosis
  ○ Botulism
• Nutritional muscular dystrophy has been reported in rabbits, but would usually be of less acute onset
  ○ Vitamin E deficiency (such as in food stored for prolonged periods) is the cause, and clinical pathological findings include elevations of cholesterol and creatine kinase

Splay leg

• True 'splay leg' is an autosomally recessive inherited condition in which rabbits at an age of a few days to several weeks

ORGAN SYSTEMS

old develop an inability to adduct their hindlimbs or, less commonly, all four limbs

- Skeletal abnormalities are found, especially in the femurs
- Affected rabbits are unable to raise their belly from the ground
- Affected animals should be culled
- Several other similar genetic musculo-skeletal abnormalities have been described which may present with similar effects
  - Occasionally, similar signs can be seen for no apparent reason in single limbs, and amputation may be a realistic option

Toxoplasmosis

- *Toxoplasma gondii* infection is rare in rabbits, but can cause ataxia, muscle tremors, paraplegia and posterior paralysis
  - As with other non-felid species, infection comes from ingesting the organism, in cat faeces, which must be more than 2 days old for the organism to be infectious
  - Contaminated bedding, grazing areas, hay and vegetables are the most likely sources
- Diagnosis of toxoplasmosis is by combination of clinical signs and serology
  - Post-mortem histopathological finding of tachyzoites and tissue cysts in the brain
  - Differentiated histologically from *Encephalitozoon cuniculi* by strong haematoxylin staining
- Treatment has to be with potentiated sulphonamides (with or without pyrimethamine) since clindamycin is highly damaging to a rabbit's GI flora
- *Neospora caninum* infection has not yet been reported in rabbits

Sarcocystis

- *Sarcocystis cuniculi* (syn *S. leporum*)
  - Parasite endemic in wild Sylvilagus rabbits in the USA
  - Transmission to domestic *Oryctolagus cuniculi* has been reported
  - The condition does not present in the acute infection, but rupture of muscle cysts causes a severe myositis

Hydrocephalus

- Hydrocephalus can occur due to an inherited defect in drainage of CSF from the brainstem, or due to either hypo- or hypervitaminosis A
- Clinical signs include circling, convulsions, opisthotonus and collapse

Rabies

- Rabbits are relatively, but not completely resistant, to rabies virus infection; in any case, bite wounds from a rabid predator are likely to be fatal before infection takes hold
  - Neurological signs such as blindness and forelimb lameness have been described following bite wounds from an infected skunk

Lead poisoning

- Lead toxicity in rabbits is usually a vague non-specific condition with signs such as anorexia, weight loss and GI stasis
  - More advanced cases may show neurological defects
- Diagnosis
  - History of access to lead-containing materials
  - Haematology may reveal characteristic basophilic stippling of RBCs
  - Radiography of the GIT may reveal metallic densities, although these may not always be present
  - Radiography of the skull may reveal metal shavings trapped between the teeth even after the GI lead has passed through

- Treatment
  - Rabbits with suspected lead posoning should be started on chelation therapy (CaEDTA 27.5 mg/kg SC q6 h for 5 days) whilst awaiting blood lead levels (>10 μg/dL is significant)
  - Further courses of chelation may be required at weekly intervals
  - Identification of the source and 'bunny proofing' are essential to prevent recurrence
- Potential sources of lead include:
  - Weights – curtain weights especially, but also fishing and diving equipment
  - Self-righting toys
  - Batteries
  - Solder – check joints of metal articles, especially cage repairs
  - Lead pellets from shotgun cartridges or air-rifles
  - Lead-based paints, varnishes and lacquers (some lead-free paints have leaded drying agents)
  - Foil covering champagne and wine corks
  - Electricians' cable clips
  - Light bulb bases
  - Linoleum and roofing felt
  - Glazed ceramics and mirror backing
  - Costume jewellery
  - Plaster and putty
  - Leaded or stained glass windows
  - Seeds for planting (coated with lead arsenate)
  - Many rubberized plastic items, e.g. rubber toys, soles of training shoes

Seizures

- Primary idiopathic epileptic disease is rare in rabbits
  - Has been reported in white furred/blue eyed breeds such as the Vienna white and the Beveren white
  - Many inherited conditions have been propagated in laboratory rabbits, and the genes for recessively inherited conditions may occasionally surface in pet or breeding animals, including those for
    - hereditary ataxia (a glycogen storage disease)
    - shaking palsy
    - paralytic tremor (similar to Parkinson's disease)
    - syringomyelia
- Seizures are more often due to:
  - Brain or meningeal lesions (see above
    - listeriosis, pasteurellosis, *Baylisascaris*, *Encephalitozoon*, etc.)
  - Metabolic toxic conditions such as ketosis and renal failure
  - Hypoxaemia associated with severe respiratory conditions
  - Heat stroke

CLINICAL NUTRITION AND GASTROINTESTINAL DISORDERS

NUTRITIONAL REQUIREMENTS OF RABBITS

'Nearly all important disease problems in rabbits are directly or indirectly related to diet.'

Jenkins (2004a)

Precise nutritional requirements for rabbits are presented in Table 3.1

- However, most vitamin/mineral deficiencies are only a clinical problem on very tightly restricted diets
- In particular, a rabbit able to perform caecotrophy should receive adequate amounts of B vitamins and vitamin K
- The biggest problem in pet rabbits is feeding sufficient fibre whilst minimizing the intake of protein, fat and carbohydrates

Table 3.1   Nutrient requirements of rabbits

Dietary component	Clinical notes
Vitamin A	Most concentrate feeds are formulated to give in the region of 10 000 iu/kg; most hay-based diets have twice that amount. Signs of deficiency include xerophthalmia, keratinization of epithelia, reproductive abnormalities (resorbtion, abortion, hydrocephalus, stillbirth) and ataxia Hepatic coccidiosis increases the requirements for vitamins A and E
Vitamin B complex	
Nicotinic acid	Synthesized from tryptophan, and deficiency can result if neither nicotinic acid nor tryptophan are present in the diet
B_6	Deficiency has been suggested as the cause of weight loss, convulsions and dermatitis
Niacin	Weight loss, diarrhoea, anorexia
Biotin	Alopecia, dermatitis
Vitamin C	Unnecessary, but no evidence of toxicity
Vitamin D	See notes. Some evidence suggests delayed mineralization in kits on deficient diets and 900 iu/kg food has been suggested as an appropriate inclusion rate Toxicity is widely reported (at 2300 iu/kg feed), resulting in mineralization of the aorta and kidney, anorexia, weight loss and infertility. Hypophosphataemia develops rather than hypercalcaemia. Eventually uraemia signals renal failure
Vitamin E/selenium	Low levels in feed have been reported to cause muscular dystrophy in youngsters fed on severely high fat diets (e.g. using cod liver oil as a supplement) Suggested requirements include 0.2–0.4 mg alpha-tocopherol/kg daily if on a 10% fat pelleted diet, or 50 mg/kg feed There is some evidence of reproductive effects Selenium may not exert the same degree of synergistic effect in rabbits as in other species
Vitamin K	Neccessary for reproduction – haemorrhagic abortions occur in deficient does, despite no clotting alterations in doe
Ca	See notes <0.2% in diet leads to spinal fractures <0.08% causes lens opacities, tetany, lowered serum total Ca Recommendations are 2 g/rabbit/day (0.6–1% of diet) during growth/pregnancy and 2.5 g/rabbit/day during lactation; pet rabbit maintenance 510 mg/day

Table 3.1 (continued)

Dietary component	Clinical notes
Phosphorus	Some poor quality hays seem deficient Increasing intake in one study from 0.07% to 0.17% gave increased growth and improved calcification NRC[a] growth diet = 0.48%
Mg	Deficiency causes decreased growth rate, hyperirritability, convulsions and death Recommended intake is 30–40 mg $MgSO_4$/100 g diet High Ca and P compete with Mg
Potassium	<0.3% leads to muscular dystrophy >0.8% gives maximum growth rates
NaCl	0.5–1% of commonly used pelleted diets Low levels lead to decreased food utilization, low milk production and possibly loss of renal concentrating ability
Iron and Cu	Deficiency of both iron and copper causes anaemia in weanlings Copper deficiency alone causes greying of black hair, decreased growth, hair loss, dry scaly skin NRC[a] growth diet gives 36 mg Fe and 2.7 mg Cu daily – these values seem well in excess of those neccessary to prevent deficiencies Copper at 400 ppm in the diet is suggested to maximize growth
Choline	Deficiencies cause decreased growth, liver damage, muscular dystrophy and haemorrhagic renal degeneration Requirement estimated at 0.13% of diet
Manganese	<0.3 mg daily causes bone deformities in weanlings 1 mg/day is suggested as the requirement
Cobalt	Small requirement for bacterial B_{12} synthesis in gut (cobalamin)

[a] National Research Council.

- Calcium and vitamin D are also important issues

Fibre
- Rabbits require high fibre levels to drive optimum gut mobility and provide the right environment for caecal microflora
- Indigestible fibre consists of particles longer than 0.5 mm
  - Stimulates GI motility
  - Provides dental wearing
- Fermentable fibre is less than 0.3 mm long
  - Provides a substrate for caecal fermentation
  - Gives caecotrophs their firm consistency
  - Provides optimum caecal pH and VFA production, preventing the proliferation of pathogenic bacteria
- Inadequate long fibre levels are associated with sluggish GI motility and increased

caecal pH, favouring clostridial and coliform overgrowth
- Inadequate fibre enables a solid food ball to be formed in the stomach, with the risk that gastric acid is unable to penetrate, leading to bacterial enteritis and caecal dysbiosis

Fat
- High fat levels are associated with rapid weight gain and high palatability, but also with rancidity of stored food, obesity and atherosclerosis

Protein
- Protein levels required vary with lifestage
  ○ Excessive levels adversely affect caecal microflora
  ○ Predispose to reduced GI motility and excessive caecotroph accumulation

Carbohydrate
- Carbohydrate requirements are low
  ○ Nearly always exceeded, sometimes massively, by proprietary foods
  ○ High quantities of simple carbohydrates lead to caecal dysbiosis and a variety of enteropathies, as well as obesity and dental disease

Selective feeding
- Selective feeding is a very important issue in considering optimum nutrition
- The overall breakdown of dietary ingredients of a feed may be absolutely perfect, but if certain elements of the food are preferred over others, then the *actual* intake of nutrients may be seriously incorrect
- In particular, the most palatable items, such as biscuit meal, flaked peas, rolled oats and maize, are often eaten almost to the exclusion of all others, which means that the *actual* diet of the rabbit is low in fibre, calcium and vitamin D, yet high in carbohydrate and protein

Practical feeding of pet rabbits
- Maximize the intake of long fibre
  ○ Grass (fresh, dried)
  ○ Hay
  ○ Fibrous leafy weeds and vegetables with moderately high calcium contents
- This can be achieved by allowing rabbits to forage naturally in gardens for grass, or bringing in plucked grass (not clippings) for house rabbits, plus vegetables (mainly leaves rather than roots)
  ○ They will also enjoy tree bark and leaves, growing tips of plants, stems and roots, of both 'weeds' and domesticated plants
  ○ In winter, increased reliance on hay and dried grass is necessary
- The use of pelleted diets should be minimized, and ideally reserved for those rabbits with high energy and protein requirements during:
  ○ Growth
  ○ Pregnancy
  ○ Lactation
  ○ It should be noted that wild UK rabbits, in the same environment as domestic pet rabbits and eating simply grass and leafy weeds, are able to breed prolifically

Pelleted foods or mixes should either be of the homogenous extruded form, or fed using a 'clean bowl' policy, i.e. ensuring that the rabbit eats all components of the mix. In any case, only tightly restricted amounts of pelleted food should be fed.

Timothy hay is believed to be the ideal type for rabbits, but is difficult to acquire reliably all year round.
- Imported US supplies are available, and small producers in the UK may be found
- Meadow hay is the next best, but can be dustier
- Abrasiveness is a factor of both grass species and age before reaping

Dietary changes

The diet of a sick rabbit should not be changed, other than to directly treat its disease state

- At this stage, eating anything is more important than attempting to force the rabbit to eat the 'correct' diet, and inducing anorexia
- Dietary changes for any rabbit should be made gradually, to avoid anorexia or abrupt caecal microflora changes

LIFESTAGE NUTRITION

Exact nutritional requirements vary with lifestage, with the main nutrients varying according to Table 3.2.

- Calcium requirements of rabbits can change with lifestage
- Generally, very high calcium content foods, e.g. alfalfa hay, should be reserved for those individuals which are growing, lactating or pregnant
- Calcium supplementation should only be used where clinically necessary

Table 3.2 Variation in rabbit nutrient requirements at several life stages

Energy requirement

Basal	40 kcal/kg plus 20 kcal per day
Reproduction	Increase by 50% for last third of pregnancy
Lactation	2–3 times maintenance by week 4 of lactation
Growth	Between 5 and 10 kcal per gram of weight gain

Protein requirements

Basal	35 g/1000 kcal
Pregnancy	42 g/1000 kcal
Lactation	50 g/1000 kcal
Growth	Initially as lactation, later dropping to maintenance by 8 months

These figures equate to protein levels of approx. 16% for growth, 20% for lactation, 14% for pregnancy and 12% for maintenance. Some 90% of ingested protein is absorbed in the small intestine

Fat requirements

Requirement is 1–3%, particularly of eicosanoid EFAs. Note that >10% fat increases palatability and weight gain, but also increases risks of atherosclerosis in older animals. Some rabbit strains get atherosclerosis even on a zero fat diet. Fat levels are increased in concentrates to decrease dustiness and crumbling of pellets. High fat levels may cause rancidity if stored for long periods

Fibre requirements

Estimated at 10–16% for lactating does; 20–26% at all other times; >10% indigestible. Increasing fibre content of pelleted diets increases their acceptability. Decreasing the fibre leads to an increase in caecal pH allowing clostridial and coliform overgrowths

ORGAN SYSTEMS

NUTRITIONAL MANAGEMENT OF THE ANOREXIC OR HOSPITALIZED RABBIT

Free choice
- Food should always be offered ad libitum to any anorexic or hospitalized rabbit
  - This food should include a selection of items the rabbit is known to enjoy
  - Bringing the rabbit's own food from home is useful
- In addition, offering good quality loose hay (e.g. Timothy) and fresh items, e.g. grass, dandelions, carrot tops, kale and other green leafy vegetation, is important
  - Shredding or chopping these can make it easier to eat them
  - The water content of such foods can be increased by dipping them in water, steaming them or sprinkling water on them, increasing palatability and water intake
- Softening the rabbits' own pelleted food, or an extruded pellet such as Burgess Excel, with water increases palatability and ease of eating, and many rabbits will accept this when they show no interest in the dry pellets
  - Some rabbits prefer such 'mash' if prepared using warm water
- Fresh water should always be provided
  - It should always be provided in a manner that is familiar to that rabbit
  - If in doubt provide water both in a bowl and a drinker
  - Bowls may be easier for post-surgical and post-dental rabbits to drink from
  - Bottled or filtered water may be better, to avoid the unpalatability of chlorinated water or water of different hardness than the rabbit is used to

Assisted or force feeding
- This is necessary in any case where the rabbit is anorexic and/or suffering from GI stasis

- Hepatic lipidosis can develop within 24 hours of cessation of feeding, and the prognosis for successful treatment of anorexia/gut stasis markedly worsens with duration
- The aim of nutritional management in such cases is to prevent protein energy malnourishment developing at a point where such requirements are *increased* (i.e. post surgery or disease) due to 'stressed starvation' or 'hypermetabolism'
  - If this is not achieved, the rabbit will start to utilize free fatty acids rather than glucose and VFAs as an energy source, leading to hepatic lipidosis and ketoacidosis
- In the early stages of anorexia, glucose alone may be sufficient
  - As anorexia progresses, protein, fat and fibre (to maintain gut motility and produce VFAs) are more important
- Short-term nutritional support, e.g. immediately post-operatively aims to provide energy in the form of glucose to prevent hypoglycaemia and mobilization of free fatty acids
- In longer-term nutrition, it is important to provide both indigestible and fermentable fibre, to drive gut motility, and provide a substrate for caecal fermentation, respectively

There are two main methods of supplementary feeding:
- Oral administration
- Administration directly into the oesophagus or stomach
  - The decision as to which method to use depends on
    — Duration of anorexia
    — Amount of food the rabbit requires
    — Response of the rabbit to the relative stresses of the two methods

Syringe
- In most cases it is simplest to administer food by mouth

○ Various feeding implements can be used, but an appropriately sized syringe is most usual

○ Some operators favour larger sizes to avoid constant refilling or changing of syringes, whereas some favour many small (e.g. 1 ml syringes) which can be more easily handled and positioned into the mouth

• Using wide nozzled syringes (or cutting the luer lock fittings off smaller syringes) allows higher fibre food to be given

• Some rabbits may accept food simply hand fed to them, especially long leafy palatable items, which can be slowly 'posted' into the rabbit's mouth

Advantages
• Technically straightforward
• With gentle restraint, in a well handled rabbit, not too stressful
• Thicker foodstuffs (i.e. with a high long fibre content) may be given, especially if wide nozzled syringes are used

Disadvantages
• Care must be taken to avoid rapid infusion resulting in inhalation pneumonia
• The rabbit must be restrained multiple times daily, which can be very stressful for some individuals
• Not suitable for cases where there has been severe facial trauma, e.g. mandibular fractures

Naso-oesophageal/nasogastric tubes
• Generally speaking, this is the only method used to enterically feed a rabbit other than by the oral route
  ○ Oesophagostomy and gastrostomy feeding tubes are not used to any degree in practice situations
• A nasogastric/naso-oesophageal tube is placed (conscious, using local anaesthetics only in the debilitated rabbit, or under sedation or anaesthesia as necessary) as in the cat

○ Tubes can easily end up passing down the trachea rather than the oesophagus
○ The head is held ventroflexed to minimize the risk of tracheal placement
— Confirm correct placement before any material is administered
— Rabbits have a very poor cough reflex, and test administration of sterile fluid is not a reliable method
— In an anaesthetized rabbit, prior endotracheal tube placement or laryngoscopic visualization of the larynx can be used to confirm oesophageal positioning of the tube
– If placed in a sedated or conscious rabbit, radiography is necessary to confirm position
• A 6–8 French size tube is suitable for the average 2.5 kg rabbit

Advantages
• Once placed, handling stress is very much reduced
• Large volumes can be administered without prolonged handling
• Once correctly placed, the risk of aspiration pneumonia is negligible, unless the rabbit is overfed
• Oral fluids and drugs can easily be administered
• Rabbits are able to eat with the tube in place

Disadvantages
• Placement requires sedation or anaesthesia in many cases
• Significant risk of tube placement in trachea
  ○ Confirmation of correct placement necessary (see above)
• Nearly all cases require an Elizabethan collar to prevent removal of the tube by the rabbit
  ○ This prevents caecotrophy and is stressful for the rabbit
• The tube diameter rarely permits the administration of a food high enough in

indigestible long fibre to drive normal GI motility
- This technique is most applicable to treatment of rabbits at severe risk of hepatic lipidosis to correct energy crises, rather than for tempting the anorexic rabbit to eat

Other enteric feeding methods
- Pharyngostomy tubes have been widely used in laboratory rabbit medicine and their use seems well tolerated
- They may have a place in longer term nutrition, especially in rabbits suffering severe head trauma
- Percutaneous endoscopic gastrostomy tubes are not well tolerated, and the procedure would predispose to GI stasis, trichobezoar formation and peritoneal adhesion formation

Total parenteral nutrition
- Long term total parenteral nutrition is not practicable in the rabbit
  - It is impossible to maintain gut motility in such a situation
  - It is unusual to use parenteral nutrition at all in rabbits
- Short term partial parenteral nutrition, aimed at providing fat and carbohydrate for energy metabolism, and protein for synthesis, may have a role to play in rabbits in severe catabolic states
  - The aim is to mirror the current metabolic condition of the liver (estimated by monitoring ketones in blood and urine) and provide mainly carbohydrate or lipid as necessary
  - In most cases of prolonged (i.e. over 3 days) anorexia, lipid is the primary substrate
  - Excessive lipid administration can lead to liver pathology, coagulopathies, thrombocytopaenia, atherosclerosis and effects on immune function
  - Provision of PPN for around 3 days is usual

- In less extreme cases (again particularly in cases involving hepatic lipidosis, pregnancy toxaemia and ketoacidosis), provision of parenteral glucose, and vitamin- and amino-acid-containing fluids such as Duphalyte (Fort Dodge Animal Health) may be beneficial

Foodstuff
- A variety of foodstuffs have been advocated for supplementary feeding in rabbits
- Proprietary liquid foodstuffs such as Critical Care Formula (VetArk) provide energy in the form of long chain carbohydrates, and are therefore perhaps more useful that simple oral rehydration fluids (e.g. Lectade, Pfizer), although the latter have their place in initial rehydration
  - These can easily be administered through almost any size tube
- Proprietary mashes such as Oxbow Critical Care for Herbivores (Oxbow), or Supreme Recovery Diet (Supreme Petfoods) make a thicker semi-liquid
  - Nutritionally these are superior as they provide long indigestible fibre particles to stimulate GI motility
  - They can be difficult or impossible to pass down all but the largest diameter tubes
- Home made diets can also be used
  - Soaked extruded rabbit pellets (e.g. Burgess Excel)
  - Powdered or tablet form alfalfa or barley grass mixed with water
  - Non-meat and dairy (preferably organic) baby food
  - Liquidized vegetation (e.g. pumpkin, carrot, grass, hay or dark green leaves, etc.)
  - Again, the thickest consistency and highest long-particle-fibre foods are not suitable for nasogastric tube feeding
- Concerns have been raised as to causing enterotoxaemia by giving a food too high in simple sugars (e.g. baby foods)

○ This does not appear to be a practical problem

○ Providing a rapidly obtainable source of energy to avoid hepatic lipidosis seems more important, with deaths in such cases nearly always being due to hepatic lipidosis, and rarely to enterotoxaemia

• Amounts required vary depending on whether the rabbit is eating any other food, how much fluid has been used to dilute the food, and the nutritional contents of the food

○ 30–5 ml/kg/day given in divided amounts every 4–8 hours is suggested

NUTRITIONAL MANAGEMENT OF SPECIFIC DISEASE STATES

Generally speaking, the advice for any disease process other than that requiring supportive feeding as above is to feed the rabbit according to the guidelines given in Practical feeding of pet rabbits, p. 108.

• There are few deviations from this general rule

• Any change in diet should be performed slowly, and the rabbit observed closely to ensure that it is actually eating the new diet, as anorexia due to dietary change can be fatal

• Any rabbit undergoing a diet change should first be given a full clinical examination, including a full dental examination

Obesity

• Weight loss should be gradual, consisting of no more than 1.5% per week

○ The rabbit should be gradually weaned off pelleted food and mixes

○ Any 'treats', e.g. bread, toast, breakfast cereals or even in some cases chocolate, should be stopped

○ The rabbit should be fed as recommended in Practical feeding of pet rabbits, p. 108, with hay, grass and dark green leafy vegetation only

• The rabbit is unlikely to become underweight if kept on such a diet long term, unless some pathological process is present

• Exercise should also be increased

Hepatic lipidosis

• This is usually as a result of anorexia

• It is vitally important to provide an easily assimilated source of glucose, either parenterally (and)/or orally, in the early stages

○ Whilst *Clostridium spiroforme* requires glucose to produce iota toxin, and therefore, in theory, provision of simple sugars should encourage this condition, this rarely seems to occur in practice, whereas lack of easily assimilated energy can encourage further development of hepatic lipidosis, with fatal consequences

• After that, it is important to provide an energy source sufficient to avoid further catabolic changes

• This will often require supplementary feeding as detailed above

• If the rabbit is overweight, once the crisis is over, weight loss, together with the treatment of any other underlying factors, is necessary

Urinary tract disorders

• 'Sludge' is postulated to be caused by a relative excess of calcium in the diet, and therefore in the urine

• The actual amount may not be excessive, and it may only be present in excess in the urine through other factors which must be addressed in conjunction with dietary change:

○ Positioning for urination

○ Mobility of the rabbit

○ Water intake

ORGAN SYSTEMS

- Reduction in calcium intake *may* be necessary
  - In general, many rabbits' diets are too low in calcium, due to selective feeding on low calcium items
  - Alfalfa can contain too much calcium for adult rabbits that are not pregnant or lactating, and should be avoided in cases of 'sludge'
  - Timothy hay and timothy based pellets are preferred to alfalfa in these cases
- The diet should be changed to one high in grass, hay and green leafy vegetables, and low in pelleted foods
- Any supplementation, unless clinically necessary for other reasons, should be withdrawn
- Feeding foods of moderate to high calcium content, which also have high levels of water and fibre (e.g. watercress, dandelion, parsley), is unlikely to add to the problem
  - See p. 117 for a list of other foods by calcium content
- Increase in water intake is beneficial in cases of urinary tract 'sludge' and urinary tract infection
  - Flavouring the water with fruit juice or cordial appeals to some rabbits, but others are deterred by the taste
    — Sticky residues may prevent the drinker nozzles from working
    — Sugar may encourage bacterial growth, so water must be changed once or twice daily
  - Provision of salt licks has been suggested to increase thirst, although at the risk of affecting electrolyte parameters
  - Syringing fluid into the rabbit by mouth daily is possible, depending on owner and rabbit compliance
  - Increasing the water content of food is easier and less stressful than administering fluid by syringe, and can be carried out by switching to fresh rather than dried vegetation, steaming or dipping hay, sprinkling water on food items, and allowing access to grazing

at night and in the early hours of the morning when dew is present
- Hardness of water depends on mineral content and has been suggested as a factor in palatability; bottled or filtered water may be preferred by some rabbits
- Some plants are believed to have a mild natural diuretic action, and it may be worth increasing the amount of these that are fed, e.g. yarrow, dandelion
  - Other plants may have a protective effect on bladder mucosa, e.g. cranberry (extract is more palatable than berries or juice)
- It is not possible (or desirable if it were) to acidify the urine of herbivores in an attempt to dissolve crystals
  - Urinary tract acidifiers have no place in the management of urinary tract disease of rabbits

Dental disease

The exact contribution of diet to dental disease is somewhat controversial, but there appear to be two main factors involved:
- The first is the relative lack of dental wear resulting from low fibre diets which are high in calories, and require little chewing
- The second is the low calcium/vitamin D content of such diets, and the resultant nutritional secondary hyperparathyroidism leads to poor dental conformation

Whether either or both of these theories are correct, the correction of the diet to the standard diet advised earlier is helpful in preventing dental disease.
- Once dental disease has started, there is permanent malformation of the teeth, that no amount of dietary change will affect
- Correcting the diet may prevent a worsening of the underlying pathology, but will not affect the malocclusion present
  - Rabbits with painful mouths as a result of tooth pathology will not be

as conducive to dietary changes, and may resist changes to diets higher in fibre that are more difficult to eat
- o Particular care is necessary in these cases to avoid compounding anorexia, and especially palatable items such as fresh grass and dandelions may be used
- The absence of incisors or even molars does not appear to prevent rabbits from eating hay, long grass or vegetables if they enjoy them
  - o Rabbits with no incisors often find it difficult to graze short vegetation effectively
  - o Rabbits with absent teeth may not be able to masticate long stranded vegetation or root vegetables, and may benefit from having these chopped into bite-sized pieces

Gastrointestinal disease
The provision of a diet with optimum fibre, fat, protein and carbohydrate levels as detailed in 'Practical feeding of pet rabbits' on p. 108 is ideal for rabbits that are prone to excessive caecotroph accumulation, GI stasis, diarrhoea and enteritis, although the immediate disease process must initially be addressed, and whilst such a diet can be offered, many of these conditions occur alongside anorexia, so supplementary feeding will be necessary, at least in the short term.

Renal disease
- Phosphate restriction may be necessary
  - o Reduce amounts of carrots, tomatoes and banana in particular
- Moderate protein levels should be fed
  - o Reduce amount of pelleted food
- Avoid dietary nephrotoxins, e.g. oxalates, found in aged dock leaves, beetroot leaves, oak leaves, for example

TOXIC PLANTS

- Note that toxicity depends on the stage of growth, the part eaten, and the state (e.g. fresh or dried)
- This list is not exhaustive
- There is some controversy over exactly how toxic plants are to rabbits, with some authorities pointing out that rabbits' lack of a vomiting reflex makes it difficult to rid themselves of ingested toxins
- Others note that rabbits appear resistant to the plant toxins contained in ragwort, deadly nightshade, laburnum and comfrey

- Agave
- All plants growing from bulbs, e.g. daffodils
- Amaryllis
- Anemones
- Antirrhinums
- Arum (lords and ladies)
- Avocado leaf
- Azalea
- Bittersweet
- Bluebell
- Boxwood
- Bracken
- Bryony
- Buttercups (although apparently small amounts dried and bundled in hay are harmless)
- Caladium
- Castor oil plant
- Celandine
- Charlock
- Chrysanthemums
- Clematis
- Cloth of gold
- Columbine
- Convolvulus
- Crocus
- Cyclamen
- Daffodil
- Dahlias
- Datura
- Delphiniums
- Dock leaves once flowers appear and leaves become woody
- Dog's mercury
- Most evergreen trees
- Fig
- Figwort
- Fool's parsley
- Foxglove

- Ground elder once the flowers appear
- Ground ivy
- Gypsophilia
- Hellebore
- Hemlock
- Henbane
- Holly
- Honeysuckle
- Horse chestnut
- Horsetails
- Hyacinth
- Iris
- Ivy berries
- Jasmine
- Jerusalem cherry
- Juniper trees
- Kingcup
- Laburnum (controversial: may be resistant)
- Laurels
- Leyland cypress
- Lilies
- Lily of the valley
- Linseed oil cake (in excess)
- Lobelia
- Love-in-a-mist
- Lupins
- Marsh marigold
- Meadow saffron
- Mistletoe
- Monkshood
- Morning glory
- Nightshades (all types)
- Oak leaves
- Oleander
- Philodendron
- Pokeweed
- Poppies
- Potato tops
- Primroses
- Privet
- Ragwort (controversial: may cause liver failure, but rabbits appear highly resistant compared to other species)
- Rhododendron
- Scarlet pimpernel
- Solomon's seal
- Speedwell
- Spindle tree
- Spurges
- Star of Bethlehem
- St John's wort
- Sumach trees
- Toadflax
- Traveller's joy
- Tulips
- Wild celery
- Wisteria
- Wood sorrel
- Yew

EDIBLE PLANTS

- Acorn
- Agrimony
- Apples
- Avens
- Bananas
- Basil
- Beech
- Beechnuts
- Berries from hawthorn and mountain ash
- Borage
- Bramble
- Broccoli
- Brussels sprouts
- Buckwheat
- Burnet
- Cabbage
- Caraway
- Carrots and carrot tops
- Cauliflower
- Celery
- Chamomile
- Chickweed
- Chinese cabbage
- Cleavers
- Clover
- Collard greens
- Coltsfoot
- Comfrey
- Coriander
- Corn marigold
- Cornsilk
- Corn spurrey
- Cow parsnip
- Cucumber
- Daisy
- Dandelions
- Deadnettles
- Dock (young leaves)
- Echinacea
- Escarole
- Fruit tree leaves, twigs
- and bark
- Garlic
- Goat's rue
- Golden rod
- Goosegrass
- Green peppers
- Ground elder (before flower buds appear)
- Groundsel
- Hawthorn berries
- Hazel
- Hogweed
- Kale
- Knapweed
- Knotgrass
- Knotted persicaria
- Lady's thumb
- Lettuce
- Lucerne
- Mallow
- Marsh mallow

- Mayweeds
- Meadow horsetail
- Melon
- Milk thistle
- Mint
- Mouse ear
- Nettles
- Oak leaves (young)
- Orache
- Oxeye daisy
- Pale smartweed
- Parsley
- Peach
- Pea pods
- Pear
- Plantains
- Pineapple
- Radish and radish tops
- Raspberry leaves
- Rose
- Sea beet
- Shepherd's purse
- Sow thistle
- Spinach
- Spring greens
- Strawberries
- Sunflower
- Thistles
- Tomato
- Trefoil
- Vetch
- Watercress
- Wild carrot
- Wild strawberry
- Willow
- Yarrow

HIGH CALCIUM CONTENT PLANTS

- Alfalfa
- Broccoli
- Carrot tops
- Chinese cabbage
- Clover
- Collard greens
- Dandelions
- Goosegrass
- Kale
- Mustard greens
- Parsley
- Shepherd's purse
- Sowthistle
- Spearthistle
- Spinach
- Turnip
- Watercress

LOW CALCIUM CONTENT PLANTS

- Apple
- Bananas
- Barley
- Beans
- Bran
- Bread
- Brussels sprouts
- Carrots
- Cauliflower
- Celery
- Cucumber
- Lettuce
- Maize
- Oats
- Peas
- Pineapple
- Sunflower seeds
- Tomato
- Wheat

ORAL DISORDERS

The oral cavity is difficult to examine fully in the conscious rabbit. The use of an auroscope allows a good, magnified view of parts of the inside of the mouth, but lesions are easily missed this way, particularly in the uncooperative rabbit. Sedation or GA is mandatory for a full clinical examination of the inside of the mouth. The use of purpose designed gags and speculae greatly assists examination. Good lighting, both bright enough and directable enough, is vital. Magnification is often necessary to spot small lesions. The use of an endoscope permits very close examination of each tooth in turn.

Teeth
Hereditary malocclusion
- Incisor malocclusion can occur as an inherited problem

ORGAN SYSTEMS

ORGAN SYSTEMS

- Autosomal recessive trait
  - Any breed or strain of rabbit
  - Particularly common in breeds with a bodyweight of less than 1.5 kg, especially Netherland dwarfs
- The relatively short maxilla leaves the incisors out of occlusion
  - Upper incisors curl laterally in a tight circle
  - Lower incisors extend directly in front
- The condition presents early in the rabbit's life
  - 3 weeks to 4 months of age
- In the initial stages, the teeth remain symmetrical and have normal enamel structure
- Treatment options
  - Regular trimming every 4 to 6 weeks
  - Surgical removal

Traumatic dental disease

- Occasionally trauma to the teeth themselves or to the jaw will result in dental abnormalities
  - Simple trauma to the incisor teeth will temporarily take them out of occlusion with resultant overgrowth of the opposing tooth
- Repeated trimming of the opposing tooth may allow occlusion to return to normal provided there is no damage to the tooth apex
- Incisor extraction may be indicated if there has been damage to the tooth apex resulting in malposition of the regrowing tooth

Acquired dental disease (ADD)

- ADD is an extremely common condition in pet rabbits, and is an underlying factor behind many other clinical processes
- ADD does not occur in wild rabbits or in rabbits housed with free access to outdoor grazing all year round
- Although genetic factors may play a part, the major influence on development and progression of ADD is diet

- Rabbits are folivores: they have evolved to consume leaves and stems, predominantly of grasses which are high in fibre and also high in calcium
- Commercially available pelleted diets can match these levels of fibre and calcium quite well and the incidence of ADD in rabbits fed on such diets is low
- Cereal based 'mix' type diets allow selective eating, and the majority of rabbits avoid the pellets (which contain the majority of the fibre and the vitamins and minerals) in favour of more palatable components such as flaked maize and peas
- The reason diet has such an effect on the development of ADD is an issue of debate
  - Some authors feel that the primary problem is a decreased rate of attrition of the continually erupting crowns because of decreased abrasiveness of the selected dietary components
  - However, recent work has pointed to an underlying metabolic bone disease resulting in decreased mineral deposition in both the teeth and the perialveolar bone
  - This also suggests that exposure to ultraviolet light may play an important part, although vitamin D metabolism in the rabbit differs significantly from that in most other species

Grading

ADD is a progressive condition which generally follows a set pattern which has been graded by Frances Harcourt-Brown as follows:

Grade 1
- Normal

Grade 2
- Root elongations and deterioration in tooth quality

○ There may be no clinical signs at this stage, and findings variably include discoloration and 'ribbing' of the enamel of the incisors, palpable bony swellings on the ventral mandibular border, epiphora due to tear duct occlusion by the incisor root

Grade 3

• Acquired malocclusion
  ○ Alterations in the position and structure of the teeth change the direction of growth and can lead to clinical malocclusion problems – teeth may impinge on tongue, lips or gums, and the resultant pain can lead to altered grooming and ingestion patterns, drooling of saliva, polydipsia and anorexia
  ○ Loosening of the teeth and widening of the periodontal space allow penetration of food material and bacteria leading to periodontal infection and abscessation

Grade 4

• Cessation of tooth growth
  ○ Progressive alteration to the structure of the tooth apices eventually results in slowing or cessation of tooth growth
  ○ At this stage, provided the rabbit can be fed a diet which it can consume without the need for chewing, the clinical condition often greatly improves as the teeth no longer grow to impinge on the gums or tongue
  ○ Periodontal abscessation is still a risk

Grade 5

• 'End-stage' dental disease
  ○ Periodontal infection results in osteomyelitis and abscessation which completely destroy the tooth apices
  ○ In some cases the inflammatory process results in fusion of the remaining tooth stump to the surrounding diseased bone

Treatment of ADD

• Where possible, attempt should be made to rectify the dietary problems which have led to the development of ADD
  ○ This can be difficult because once ADD is clinically present (grade 3 and above) the altered occlusion and loosening of the teeth make normal consumption of grass, hay and leafy vegetables more difficult
  ○ Supplementation with calcium and vitamin D, and access to unfiltered sunlight (or artificial ultraviolet light) should be considered in rabbits which are unable to consume a normal diet
• Treatment of clinical ADD is palliative rather than curative
  ○ The alterations to the structure of the teeth and the periodontal structures are permanent and cannot be restored to the original conformation
• Treatment usually needs to be repeated, often as frequently as every 6–12 weeks for the rest of the rabbit's life (possibly less often if the condition progresses to grade 4 – see above)

There are two main aims of treatment of ADD:

• The first is to restore the rabbit to a state in which it is comfortable
  ○ This can be achieved under GA by removing spikes or spurs on the teeth which are rubbing against the gums or tongue, and where necessary by the use of NSAIDs
  ○ Whilst some authors find the use of nail clippers or similar instruments effective, the shattering effect that these can have on the teeth potentially causes fracture lines into the tooth pulp cavity with resultant pain and possibly infection
  ○ The alternative is to use a dental burr or similar mechanical instrument to cut the teeth with more control, but

ORGAN SYSTEMS

when using such instruments it is essential to have excellent exposure of the oral cavity, where possible using illumination and magnification, to ensure that surrounding soft tissues are not damaged

- The second aim is to attempt to reduce the risk of further damage or infection to the tooth apices
  - Elongated and loosened tooth crowns cannot exert the normal rasping action even if they remain in occlusion
  - Reducing the crowns of these teeth to the normal length, or even shorter, reduces the leverage applied to them (reducing the risk of food material and bacteria entering the periodontal space) and so may help to reduce the risk of periodontal abscessation
  - There are concerns, however, that shortening the teeth in this way may take them out of occlusion and therefore prevent the rabbit from consuming a normal diet
  - Teeth which have become severely loosened should be extracted via an oral approach

Oral abscesses due to laceration by spurs

- Some abscesses form where there has been chronic laceration of the buccal mucosa by spikes or spurs that are formed on the overgrown crowns of the teeth
  - In these cases treatment is by correction of the underlying tooth deformity, expression or curettage of as much pus as possible and antibiosis
  - The prognosis in these cases is generally reasonable provided repeated dentistry is performed to prevent regrowth of the spur
  - See Soft tissue lesions below for treatment of abscesses

Abscesses due to tooth root penetration

- Abscesses associated with the roots of the teeth are far more difficult to deal with
  - Where possible, the tooth involved should be identified and extracted, although once periodontal infection, osteomyelitis and abscessation have developed there are often several tooth roots involved in the abscess
  - Teeth can be extracted either via an oral approach, or during surgery on the abscess itself
  - See Soft tissue lesions below for treatment of abscesses

Soft tissue lesions
Lips
Myxomatosis

- Oedema of the lips and facial skin occurs in myxomatosis
- Diagnosis is based on the almost pathognomonic clinical appearance, with definitive diagnosis on electron microscopy
- There is no specific cure for myxomatosis, although supportive care and good nursing may enable recovery in some mildly affected rabbits (see Myxomatosis, p. 188)

Rabbit syphilis

- *Treponema cuniculi* affects the mucocutaneous junctions of the face
- The genitals are also often affected, as with myxomatosis, but there is not generally oedema, and it is usually possible to differentiate the two diseases just on physical appearance
- Dark field microscopy or silver stains identify the organism
- *T. cuniculi* is sensitive to a number of antibiotics
- See also Treponemiasis, p. 193

Trauma to the lips and tongue

- Physical, chemical or thermal
- There is often a history of fighting, damaged jagged water drinkers or wire, or access to caustic chemicals
- Treatment generally involves providing supportive care, including analgesia to minimize the risk of anorexia
- Supportive fluids and supplementary feeding may be necessary if the rabbit is struggling to eat

Perioral abscessation

Although occasionally associated with bite wounds or foreign body penetrations, the vast majority of abscesses around the facial area of the rabbit are associated with acquired dental disease

- Loosening of the teeth and widening of the periodontal space allow food materials and oral bacteria to penetrate into the periodontal area
- A particular risk factor for abscessation occurs when elongations of the apices of the teeth result in penetration of the perialveolar bone, for instance when the tooth apex reaches the periosteum or where the apices of two teeth meet
  - These penetrations occur in very predictable positions
- The oral flora of the rabbit is similar to that of other species in that a high proportion of bacteria present are anaerobic
  - Consequently, perioral abscessation of rabbits is not (as is commonly perceived) likely to be due to *Pasteurella* infection, and fluoroquinolones (although currently licensed for use in rabbits in the UK) are not a good first line choice of antibacterial drug

The general aim in most tooth root abscess cases is palliation and long term control of the abscess, rather than complete cure; rabbits which maintain good quality of life but which have to be on intermittent or continuous antibiotic treatment should be regarded as successful cases, not failures.

When considering a surgical approach to rabbit abscesses it is important to appreciate the difference from abscesses in dogs or cats

- Rabbit pus tends to form into a thick adherent paste which does not lend itself well to lancing and drainage
- The majority of the active infection is within the capsule of the abscess, not within the pus itself
  - This means that simple drainage and flushing as would be standard for a cat abscess will not be effective in the rabbit

Management of perioral abscesses must be tailored to the individual case, but in general there are three main approaches:

Palliative medical management

- In many cases the abscess itself does not cause the rabbit pain or suffering
- It may be possible to stabilize or reduce the size of an abscess simply by using long courses of antibiosis
- Where possible, samples of both pus and abscess capsule should be taken and submitted for bacteriology and sensitivity testing before beginning antibiotic courses
- The following surgical management regimes are often aimed at reducing the size of an abscess to allow palliative medical management a better chance of success

Closed management

- If the tooth involved in the abscess can be identified and removed, and the abscess and its surrounding capsule can be surgically excised, then it may be possible to suture the skin closed and a permanent cure immediately effected

ORGAN SYSTEMS

- Implantation of various antibiotic substances at the site of the abscess (antibiotic impregnated polymethylmethacrylate beads, calcium hydroxide paste, antibiotic powder) may increase the chances of success

Open management
- In many cases complete excision of the abscess capsule is not possible
  - Because it is so extensive
  - Because it involves major vessels or nerves
  - Because it merges with osteomyelitic bone
- In these cases the abscess should be opened and pus removed, and as much of the surrounding infected tissue removed as is possible
- The remaining abscess cavity can then be sutured to the skin, allowing access to the remainder of the cavity for cleansing, flushing and topical therapy
- Various topical agents can be used to aid in removal of purulent debris and to control infection:
  - Creams and pastes, e.g. Flamazine (Smith and Nephew), Fucidin (Leo), Dermisol (Pfizer)
  - Wound treatment agents, e.g. Intrasite (Smith and Nephew), Nu-gel (Johnson and Johnson)
  - Agents such as concentrated sugar solution or honey ('Manuka' honey seems a particularly effective choice)

Iatrogenic soft tissue injuries
- Damage to the buccal cavity can occur when carrying out dental treatment
- The use of rasps is commonly associated with damage to the major blood vessel at the fauces on each side
  - This can cause severe, occasionally life threatening, haemorrhage, and it is difficult to achieve haemostasis
  - In addition, blood can be inhaled and block the trachea in rabbits that are not intubated

- This is usually an acute episode, and so the history of known iatrogenic trauma is sufficient to arrive at a diagnosis
- Pressure applied via a swab held in artery forceps, or haemostats applied directly, is usually sufficient to achieve haemostasis
  - It may take some time for bleeding to stop
- Bipolar radiosurgery or proprietary haemostatic agents, e.g. Emovet (Nelson Veterinary), HemaBlock (Abbott Ltd), can also be useful
- Suturing of the tear may be indicated once haemostasis has been achieved, but requires good positioning, exposure, magnification and illumination to perform
- The use of dental burrs can also be associated with trauma
  - Although these may occasionally contact the medial aspect of the buccal mucosa, or the gum to either side of the tooth, it is rare for them to cause the injury described above
    - Such 'brushing' injuries are usually minor
  - However, it is possible for the burr to catch the loose frenulum under the tongue, which rapidly wraps itself around the burr and tears the tissue
    - This bleeds extensively, but a combination of haemostasis as above, and the suturing of the tear produced is usually sufficient to control bleeding and prevent food entrapment in the space produced
- Analgesia and systemic antibiosis are required in such cases, with supportive feeding if necessary

Uraemic stomatitis
- This may occur in rabbits in renal failure
- The clinical signs usually include anorexia, weight loss, drooling and PU/PD, and can be mistaken for, or can occur at the same time as, dental disease

- Ulcerated lesions are visible, usually on the buccal mucosa
- There may or may not be concurrent dental pathology, but blood tests for renal disease should be carried out before anaesthetizing the rabbit
- Diagnosis is based on elevated renal parameters (see Urinary tract disease, p. 150)
- Treatment
  - Assessment and management of the underlying renal disease, if possible
  - Management of any co-existing dental disease
  - Supportive care
    - fluids
    - supplementary nutrition
- The use of analgesia should be undertaken with care, as steroids and NSAIDs may worsen the existing renal disease
  - Opioids may be a useful alternative
- Prognosis varies with the severity of the renal insufficiency

Oral viral papillomas
- Small virally induced papillomas (up to 5 mm in diameter) may occur
  - They may be multiple and most commonly appear on the ventral surface of the tongue
  - They are usually self limiting within a few weeks, but some may persist for months
- Once recovered, rabbits are believed to be resistant to future infection
- No treatment is generally required

Other masses
- Tumours and granulomatous reactions to tooth impingement or foreign bodies
  - Particularly laryngeal granulomata
- Whilst relatively much rarer than in the cat, oral tumours may be under-reported
  - On gross appearance it can be impossible to distinguish them from chronic inflammation resulting from tooth

crown trauma or reactions to foreign body entrapment alongside teeth
- Biopsy and histopathology are necessary to arrive at a definitive diagnosis and prognosis
  - Although the presence of foreign material inside the lesion may increase the suspicion that it is responsible, it may be an incidental finding
- Resection or biopsy of such lesions is complicated by their friable nature, and care should be taken to avoid inhalation of blood
  - Haemostasis is as above
- Supportive nutrition and fluids may be necessary, and antibiosis given as necessary
- Analgesia is advised, both on welfare grounds and to avoid precipitating anorexia

OESOPHAGEAL DISORDERS

Oesophageal disease is extremely rare in the rabbit. The very well developed cardiac sphincter of the rabbit stomach prevents vomiting or regurgitation in all but the most extreme cases. Rabbits do not generally eat items of the correct diameter to lodge in the oesophagus, given their small oral cavity and diligent chewing actions. They do not chase sticks either, and so trauma to the oesophagus is usually limited to severe predator attacks or involvement in abscesses within the neck.

Regurgitation
- Rare, but can occur in the final stages of disease states causing gastric hypomotility
  - Most common cause is mucoid enteropathy
- Fluid overflow from the stomach can be regurgitated and inhaled, leading to death by inhalation pneumonia
- Diagnosis is on a reliable history of regurgitation

- Must be differentiated from the more common dropping of food from the mouth
- Inhalation pneumonia usually diagnosed at post-mortem examination
- Treatment in the late stages is likely to be unrewarding
- Treatment of idiopathic vomiting/regurgitation (occasionally reported) has centred on symptomatic therapy and preventing the rabbit from eating large amounts of food rapidly

Oesophageal foreign body

- Unlikely to occur as rabbits usually chew their food thoroughly and do not tend to swallow large chunks of food (e.g. carrots)
- Could occur in rabbits with voracious appetites, which are in competition to eat food rapidly with other, perhaps more dominant, rabbits
- May be more likely in rabbits that are missing a number of molars and are fed on whole or coarsely chopped root vegetables
- Diagnosis is on clinical signs:
  - Inability to swallow food
  - Drooling
  - Evidence of a foreign body on palpation or radiographic/endoscopic examinations
- Dental disease remains the most likely differential, and should be eliminated first
- Treatment involves removal of the material, either by endoscopic or surgical means
- Oesophageal mural abscesses may result from foreign body ingestion or other perforation of the oesophageal mucosa
  - These are likely, as in other species, to be challenging to treat, and manage post-operatively
  - Prevention involves cutting food into smaller pieces and avoiding hyper-competitive feeding situations

- Abscesses elsewhere in the neck may involve the oesophagus, causing extra-luminal obstructions
  - These are likely to be identified in the same way, and treatment will involve surgical exploration and attempted removal of the abscess, or at least removal of the occluding part of the abscess and capsule
  - This may be unrewarding

Oesophageal trauma

- Could occur as a result of predator trauma, where the rabbit is seized by the neck
- Generally other injuries sustained at the time are likely to be more serious:
  - Cervical dislocation
  - Vascular injuries
- Diagnosis is based on identification of damage on exploration of wounds, or endoscopic evaluation of the oesophagus, but may emerge later, when oesophageal strictures or granulomatous lesions/abscesses develop at the site of injury
  - The latter is likely to present as an oesophageal obstruction, and can be evaluated by radiography, endoscopy and surgical exploration
- Treatment depends on the duration of time since the injury, with fresh wounds easier to manage
- Abscessation/granulomatous lesions are likely to prove unrewarding to resect and repair

GASTRIC DISORDERS

- The rabbit has the largest stomach relative to body size of any mammal, and a well-developed cardiac sphincter
- These factors, combined with the poor intrinsic motility of the rabbit stomach and the often incorrect diet, contribute to make gastric disorders very common in the rabbit

- Trichobezoars, 'hairballs' or 'furballs' are no longer thought to be a cause of gastric stasis
- Whilst solid mats of fur can cause acute obstruction, moulted and ingested fur is a normal part of the stomach contents, and a hard mass of fur is a consequence, not a cause, of gastric stasis
- In the normal rabbit the stomach is hardly, or not at all, palpable
- There is always some food in the stomach, regardless of how long the rabbit has been fasted

Minimum diagnostic database

History
- Age
- Sex
- Entire or neutered?
- Single or group housed rabbit?
- Details of other rabbits kept with this one
- Detailed history of lifestyle, environment and diet including:
  - Foods offered
  - Foods eaten
  - Any history of foreign body ingestion
  - Any recent changes to diet
  - Any recent changes to environment
  - Any history of other disease, e.g. dental problems

Physical examination
- Full clinical examination, paying particular attention to oral cavity and abdomen
- Full oral/dental examination
- Abdominal palpation, auscultation and percussion

Further diagnostics and prognostic indicators
- Full haematology and biochemistry
- Survey abdominal radiographs and abdominal ultrasonography as necessary
- Dental examination under sedation or GA, and skull radiography

Prognosis
- Dependent on cause
- Only with a diagnosis, or at least the exclusion of some diagnoses, can the prognosis be determined
- If the trigger can be pinned down to a single event or problem that can be treated or avoided in future, then the long-term prognosis is excellent
- If the gut stasis goes hand in hand with, for example, chronic dental pain, especially if, as a result, the rabbit is unable or unwilling to eat high fibre food items, then recovery in the short term is dependent on treating that condition, and recurrence is very likely
- Duration of stasis
  - The longer the rabbit has not been eating or passing faeces, the more dehydrated and impacted the gut contents will be
  - Eventually, permanent and irreversible ileus will develop
  - With increasing time, recovery is less likely, and it will require a longer and more intensive course of treatment to achieve success
  - If acute obstructive lesion, prompt surgery is vital

Acute gastric disorders

Gastritis
- Bacterial gastritis in adult rabbits is very uncommon
  - Given the gastric pH of 1–2, bacteria do not generally survive
  - Toxin ingestion can lead to gastritis
  - Bacterial infections, e.g. colibacillosis, are much more common in pre-weaned rabbits where the gastric pH is higher
  - Normally the presence of naturally occurring fatty acids in the dam's milk prevents such infection
- Gastric pH can rise to 3–7 in adult rabbits with diarrhoea

ORGAN SYSTEMS

- Clinical signs in pre-weaning rabbits can include profuse watery diarrhoea, depression, anorexia
- Diagnosis is usually at post-mortem examination, with the abdomen stained yellow inside and the stomach full of undigested milk
  - Treatment with high doses of antibiotics selected on the basis of culture and sensitivity (with enrofloxacin being a good first choice for initial treatment) may help in some cases, but mortality approaches 100%
- Healthy adult rabbits have a sterile small intestine, as microorganisms are destroyed by the acidic pH of the stomach
- Healthy pre-weaning rabbits also have a sterile stomach and intestine, due to the presence of a large protective milk curd clot
- An antimicrobial fatty acid, produced in the rabbit's stomach from a substrate in the doe's milk, prevents microbial colonization
- Rabbits that do not receive mother's milk, or are in the post-weaning period, are at risk of bacterial gastritis and small intestinal infection

Gastric dilatation
Gastric stasis
- Gastric stasis should be divided into obstructive and non-obstructive disorders, which, broadly speaking, are treated surgically and medically, respectively
- Obstructive ileus is generally an acute situation
  - Non-obstructive disorders are covered under Chronic gastric disorders, p. 127. They should generally be considered a medical condition, and few cases respond to surgical intervention unless there is an intra- or extraluminal obstruction of the GIT

Obstructive ileus is typified by:
- Sudden onset (over less than 48 hours), leading to a severely moribund rabbit
- The stomach may be felt as a tympanic or firm, doughy distended mass in the left cranial abdomen
- Rabbits may be found acutely dead with this condition, often due to pyloric or small intestinal obstruction
- A sudden cessation in faecal pellet production
- Moderate to severe depression
- Marked to severe abdominal pain and guarding, with a hunched posture and reluctance to move
- Shock and moderate to severe dehydration
- Marked fluid and gas distension anterior to the site of the obstruction and bubbles of gas rather than a 'halo' in the stomach on radiography
- Fluid can build up posterior to the obstruction
- In particular, the caecum can become distended with fluid
- A large gas-filled stomach can indicate a pyloric obstruction

The initial presentation of non-obstructive ileus is usually different, and characterized as follows:
- Slow, insidious onset
- Gradual decrease in the size of faecal pellets and the frequency of their production
- Faecal pellets may also change in shape, becoming misshapen and pitted looking
- There may be a craving for high fibre items, not necessarily digestible ones, such as wood, paper, wallpaper, cardboard
- Normal hydration to moderate dehydration
- Normal demeanour at first, becoming gradually depressed and developing abdominal pain later

- Impacted material in the stomach and caecum on radiography
- There may be a 'halo' of gas around the stomach contents
- Gaseous distension develops as stasis continues, with fluid contents present in the gut in the latter stages
- Gas may be present throughout the GIT

Presentation similar to either acute or chronic gastric stasis may also be seen in mucoid enteropathy.

- Distension occurs more gradually than with foreign body obstruction.

Treatment options are detailed under Chronic gastric disorders below.

Acute obstructive ileus
- **This is an acute surgical emergency**
- The pylorus is one of the main sites for GI obstruction with foreign bodies
- Typical items include:
  - Thick mats of fur ingested intact from the feet of the rabbit or its companions
  - Clay-based clumping cat litter
  - Carpet material
  - Corn cob litter
  - Locust bean seeds
  - Corn pips
  - Dried peas
- Clinical signs are similar to those of the 'acute abdomen' in other species
  - Abdominal pain and bloating
  - Radiographic evidence of blockage
  - Debility, depression, anorexia, lethargy and collapse may be seen
  - The abdomen may feel bloated if gas build-up is present, or doughy if intestinal rupture has taken place
- Diagnosis is by identification of blockage on radiography
- Treatment involves stabilization of the rabbit for surgery with shock doses of IV or IO fluids, analgesia and antibiosis, followed by urgent exploratory laparotomy to identify and remove the blockage, and resect or repair the area of obstruction

- Gastric decompression by stomach tube may be useful in reducing bloat before surgery
- As in the GDV complex in dogs, this may have serious effects on circulation by itself, and decompression can aid in stabilization of the patient
- Needle puncture should be avoided due to the serious risk of gastric rupture and peritonitis
- Many cases will have progressed too far for even the most heroic intervention to save them
- Gastrotomy for chronic gastric stasis is generally not indicated
- There may be very occasional cases where a mass of gastric contents have become dehydrated, there is no response to medical treatment, and surgery is indicated
  - These cases carry a poor prognosis, even after apparently successful surgery, due to concurrent hepatic lipidosis

Gastric rupture
This is a common post-mortem finding in rabbits, but it usually occurs some time after death as a result of gas build-up within the stomach as fermentation of the ingesta takes place.

It may take place ante mortem in cases of gastric hypomotility, especially if over enthusiastic feeding and abdominal massage have been carried out.

It may occur subsequent to ulceration.

Chronic gastric disorders
Neoplasia
- Gastric adenocarcinoma and leiomyo-sarcoma have been reported
- Intra-abdominal local spread of uterine adenocarcinomas may occur
- Presenting signs depend on the exact site and size of the tumour
- Possible clinical signs include:
  - Anorexia, weight loss
  - Abdominal pain

- ○ Abdominal enlargement
- ○ Ascites
- ○ Cessation of faecal production
- A palpable cranial abdominal mass may be noted

Diagnosis
- Abdominal radiography and ultrasound examination
- Definitive diagnosis is on exploratory laparotomy or laparoscopy, biopsy and histopathology

Prognosis
- Guarded, as surgical resection is rarely practicable in this location in the rabbit

Abscessation
Abscess formation associated with penetrating foreign bodies (akin to traumatic reticuloperitonitis in cattle) is extremely rare. Rabbits rarely eat items sharp enough to penetrate the stomach wall. However, abscesses can develop anywhere following local trauma and bacteraemia from infection elsewhere in the body, and are a differential for neoplasia. Symptoms, diagnosis, treatment and prognosis are as above.

Gastric ulceration
Gastric ulceration is a common complication in any chronic GI disorder. Stress, poor diet, renal insufficiency and ingested toxins may also cause gastric ulceration.
- Presenting signs include abdominal pain and anorexia
- Definitive diagnosis
  - ○ Identification by endoscopic examination or laparotomy/laparoscopy
- Treatment
  - ○ Removal of causative factors, e.g. by reducing stress, dietary improvement, treatment of other GI disorders
  - ○ Symptomatic treatment with H_2 blockers, e.g. ranitidine

Stomach worms
- *Graphidium strigosum*; rare in pet rabbits
- Red, 1–2 cm long
- Attached to stomach lining
- In large numbers can cause blood loss and death
- Treatment with fenbendazole or ivermectin

Treatment of chronic, non-obstructive gastrointestinal stasis
- The initiating cause, if any can be identified, must be treated

Antibiotics
- Controversial
- Gut microbial population is likely to be abnormal enough at this time, without potentially disrupting it further
  - ○ However, may not make the situation worse
  - ○ May cover against secondary or opportunist bacterial infections, e.g. *Pasteurella* pneumonia
- If antibiotics are used, it is best to select one unlikely to have adverse effects on gut microbial populations, such as potentiated sulphonamides, tetracyclines or fluroquinolones
  - ○ If clostridial overgrowth in the gut is suspected, there is then a specific reason to use an antibiotic effective against that organism, e.g. metronidazole
- Inappropriate use of antibiotics can cause alterations in gut flora
  - ○ This can affect caecal motility, and thus actually initiate gut stasis
  - ○ Avoid penicillins, cephalosporins and especially lincosamides
  - ○ Parenteral antibiotics are less likely to be associated with problems than orally administered ones

Laxatives
- Controversial
- May assist in lubricating the passage of gut material, e.g. small hair mats

- However, may coat the gastric mass of ingesta and fur and prevent it being hydrated and broken down
- In conjunction with fluids they may help to soften and hydrate gastric contents
- Bulk laxatives that absorb water could further dehydrate both the gut contents and the rabbit itself, and should be avoided

Enemas
- These are suggested in some texts, to hydrate the distal gut
- Enemas are stressful and not without risk (the rectal and colonic wall of rabbits is extremely thin compared to that of cats and dogs), and their use is generally not advised

Enzymes, e.g. papain and bromelin
- These are found in fresh pineapple juice and contact lens protein-removing formulae
- Their use is suggested in some, particularly older, texts
- Experimentally they have not been shown to dissolve fur, and since the fur is rarely the actual problem anyway, their use is not advisable
- If they work at all, it is probably as a source of fluid and energy (in the case of pineapple juice) rather than via specific effects

Appetite stimulants
- Anything acting as an appetite stimulant may help, and is unlikely to do any harm
- Anabolic steroids, B vitamins and herbal ingredients, such as fennel, coriander and parsley, have been suggested
- B vitamins may be useful in cases where the rabbit is unable, for whatever reason, to practise caecotrophy
- Glucocorticoids should be avoided

Vitamin C
- Requirements for ascorbic acid increase during stress
- May not be necessary, as rabbits manufacture their own vitamin C
- May help prevent iota-like toxaemia

Abdominal massage
- Gentle abdominal massage to promote passage of ingesta and relief of gas accumulation
- Risk of gut perforation, especially if used in obstructive cases
- Massage pillows provide gentle vibration and rabbits can sit or lie on them
  - This may be safer and less stressful than manual massage

Exercise
- Immobility is likely to further inhibit gut motility
- Providing a large space to hop around in may help
- Encouragement to exercise is beneficial

Simethicone (Infacol, Forest Laboratories)
- May be useful in reducing excessive gas production, and the often severe pain associated with this

Cholestyramine resin (Questran, Bristol-Myers-Squibb)
- To absorb clostridial toxins
- It absorbs fluid, so should be given with concurrent fluid therapy
- May be useful if clostridial overgrowth is suspected, for example following use of some antibiotics

H_2 receptor antagonists, e.g. cimetidine, ranitidine
- With GI stasis, stress, and concurrent use of non-steroidals, there is the potential for gastric ulceration to develop
- These drugs may have a place, especially with longer-term cases
- Some evidence that these also have some GI prokinetics qualities

Probiotics

- Controversy about whether these products survive the stomach pH of 1–2 intact
- Many contain species of bacteria, especially *Lactobacillus* spp., not found in the normal rabbit gut
- Easily added to nutritional and fluid support mixtures
- Caecotrophs from a healthy rabbit are another option, but require a donor rabbit to be prevented from caecotrophy, usually by placing a buster collar, and require the caecotroph to be consumed intact

Analgesia

- Vital
  - Pain is a common cause of stasis, and if not present to start with, will compound the problem
  - Opioids and NSAIDs can be used individually or in combination
  - There is a potential risk of opioids slowing gut motility, but there is little evidence of this in practice
  - Peri-operative analgesia in rabbits is mandatory for any procedure that has the potential to cause any degree of discomfort

Gastrointestinal prokinetics

- Metoclopramide acts primarily centrally and on the foregut, and cisapride on the hindgut
- Cisapride is the most useful generally
- In combination the two drugs have a synergistic effect
- Cisapride may take longer to take effect, so concurrent use of metoclopramide at least to start with, is useful
  - Cisapride is currently out of production and likely to be unavailable in the near future
  - It is to be hoped that suitable analogues of this drug will become available

- Use of motility stimulants in obstructive ileus is contraindicated

Nutritional support

- Vital
- See Nutritional management of the anorexic or hospitalized rabbit, p. 110

Fluid therapy

- The aim is to rehydrate both the gut contents and the rabbit itself
  - Choice of routes depends on the degree of dehydration, the general state of the rabbit, and the willingness of the rabbit to accept fluids by different routes
- Oral fluids are sufficient in the early stages, but rabbits will not usually accept large quantities by this route without stress
  - They are probably the best way to get fluid into the gut, and help to hydrate and soften the gut contents
- Subcutaneous fluids are easily administered, in sizeable volumes
  - Addition of hyaluronidase at 150 iu/l of fluid speeds up their distribution from the SC space
  - In the shocked rabbit, with decreased tissue perfusion, even with hyaluronidase, they may be absorbed too slowly to have an effect
- Intravenous fluids can be given via an IV catheter placed in the marginal ear vein, which is usually well tolerated
- Intraosseous fluids can be given via an IO needle placed in the proximal humerus, tibial crest or proximal femur
  - This method has a similar rate of uptake to the IV route, but is available in even the severely shocked rabbit or those too small for IV access
- Intraperitoneal fluids are another option, and provide a rapidly available fluid bolus
  - They may have an additional benefit in bathing the fusus coli, but there is the risk of perforation of the gut

SMALL INTESTINAL DISORDERS

With the exception of coccidiosis, small intestinal disorders are relatively uncommon in the rabbit. Few microorganisms survive transit through the stomach of the adult rabbit, and the stomach and the large intestine are the main sites of GI motility disorders. Small intestinal transit should be approximately 40–80 minutes in the normal rabbit.

Intestinal coccidiosis

(See also Coccidiosis, p. 179.)
- Main sites of infection are jejunum, ileum and caecum
- There are 11 species of intestinal coccidia
- They vary greatly in their pathogenicity, and the site of their pathologic effect
- The most commonly identified species in clinical disease are *Eimeria perforans*, *E. magna*, *E. media* and *E. irresidua*
- Clinical infections can occur at any age, but are most common in young, growing rabbits, partly because one of the most important clinical signs (stunted growth) is only evident at this age
- Clinical signs can occur before oocysts are evident in the faeces

Clinical signs
- Stunting is most important
- Mild intermittent diarrhoea, with or without mucus or blood
- Weight loss
- Dehydration
- Secondary bacterial infections
- Intussusception
- Rectal prolapse
- Death

Post-mortem findings
- Inflammation, ulceration and haemorrhage of intestinal epithelium
- Site of lesions dependent on species involved

Definitive diagnosis
- Difficult, as clinical signs are similar to those of colibacillosis and other enteric diseases
- Also, coccidia are often present alongside other infections as a subclinical infestation
- Demonstration of high numbers of oocysts in faeces or intestinal contents, or confirmation of moderately high numbers of a recognized pathogenic species, ideally in conjunction with lesions in sites typical of that species, are required for definitive diagnosis

Treatment
- Robenidine, sulpha drugs, clopidol, toltrazuril and amprolium are all effective against intestinal coccidia
- Sulpha drugs have the advantage of providing some effect against secondary bacterial infections that may occur alongside coccidiosis

Prevention
- Oocysts require 2 days to sporulate in faeces
  - Hence infective oocysts do not occur in caecotrophs
- Preventing access to faeces over 2 days old is therefore effective in avoiding a build-up of pathogenic numbers
  - This can be achieved by the use of wire flooring (although this has strong negative welfare implications), deep litter systems (where heat and ammonia destroy the oocysts, though these systems are bad for respiratory health), or diligent hygiene

Foreign body impaction
- GI obstructions can also occur at the pyloroduodenal angle and the sacculus rotundus in the small intestine, as well as in the stomach
- The causes, diagnosis, prognosis and treatment options for GI foreign body

ORGAN SYSTEMS

obstruction are described in Oesophageal disorders, p. 123 and Gastric disorders, p. 124

Small intestinal microbial changes
Enteritis
- Rare in adults
  - The bacterial content of the small intestine is minimal due to the sterilizing effect on ingesta of passage through the very acidic stomach
  - In some cases, large masses of food, which are too densely packed to enable acid penetration to their core, may introduce pathogenic bacteria
    — May occur in large and/or greedy rabbits
- Reduced GI motility may delay the passage of ingesta to the caecum, leading to bacterial proliferation in the small intestine

Bacterial pathogens
- *Escherichia coli*
- Clostridia
- *Yersinia pseudotuberculosis*
  - Necrosis of Peyer's patches seen
- *Lawsonia intracellularis*
  - Proliferative ileitis (+/− enteritis)
  - Treatment challenging, as resistant to many antibiotics
    — Macrolide antibiotics (severely toxic to rabbits) are the most effective
    — Some success has been reported with chloramphenicol
    — Fluroquinolones given for at least 2 weeks may also be effective

Viral pathogens
- Rotaviruses (see Large intestinal disorders, p. 133)

Plant toxins
- May lead to enteritis

Cryptosporidium cuniculi
- Especially the ileum and jejunum

- May cause transitory diarrhoea in unweaned rabbits
- Unlikely to be significant in adult rabbits
- Self-limiting but slows growth markedly
- Organisms can be detected on ileal or jejunal smears or histopathology
- ELISA may be useful in detecting cases showing false negatives on microscopy
- *NB*: Possibly *zoonotic* in immune suppressed humans

Inflammatory conditions
- Rare
- Possibly immune mediated
- Possibly associated with post-ovaro-hysterectomy adhesions

Neoplasia, abscessation or extra-intestinal constriction
Primary neoplasia
- Intestinal leiomyoma
- Intestinal leiomyosarcoma
- Sacculus rotundus papilloma

If total removal and resection of primary neoplasia can be carried out prognosis is good.

Secondary neoplasia
- Secondary local intra-abdominal spread from uterine adenocarcinoma can occur
- Metastasis of distant neoplasia is rare

Extra-intestinal constriction
- Abdominal mass
  - Neoplasia
  - Abscess
  - Adhesion
  - Cystic calculi, etc.
- Any intra-abdominal mass causing constriction of the small intestine has the potential to cause partial or complete obstruction
- Intra-abdominal neoplasia (in particular uterine adenocarcinoma) may have such

an effect either by virtue of the size of the primary lesion, or local spread

- Intra-abdominal abscessation is not uncommon
- Infection, haemorrhage or trauma within the abdomen can very readily lead to adhesions in the rabbit
  - Abdominal surgery, e.g. ovario-hysterectomy, is probably the most common cause, but other surgery, intra-abdominal bleeding or peritonitis can also occur
- These can cause extraluminal narrowing of any part of the GIT, gas and ingesta accumulation, and contribute to or cause GI stasis

All of the above create similar clinical signs.
- Anorexia, weight loss, lack of faecal output may be seen
- There may be abdominal enlargement, ascites and abdominal pain
- The mass(es) may be palpable, or identified on abdominal radiography or ultrasonography
- Diagnosis is on laparotomy or laparoscopy and visualization of the mass
- Needle aspirates may conclusively diagnose abscesses, and biopsy and histopathology may be required to definitively diagnose neoplasia or chronic inflammatory changes
- Treatment is by surgical resection of the mass, and disentrapment or resection of the affected intestine, as necessary, if possible
- Complete surgical excision may not be possible, and the prognosis depends on the type and extent of the lesion

Intussusception
- Usually a sequel to enteric irritation (enteritis, foreign body)
- Similar presenting signs to that of a foreign body
- Usually with a palpable tubular mass at the site of the intussusception

- Usually seen in juvenile rabbits
- Stabilization and surgical correction are indicated
- Correction of the underlying problem is necessary
- Resection of gut may be required
- Prognosis is often poor, and worsens considerably with the duration of the intussusception

LARGE INTESTINAL DISORDERS

The rabbit's caecum is relatively the largest of any mammal. It consists of 40% of the volume of the GIT. The colon, under the neurological control of the fusus coli, is responsible for the separation of fermentable material from indigestible fibre. In the 'hard faeces phase' fibre is passed straight through and expelled as hard faeces. Digestible components and fluids are passed by retrograde peristalsis back up the colon and into the caecum for fermentation. In the 'soft faeces phase' which usually occurs in the early hours of the morning, caecotrophs are formed and eliminated by the colon, to be ingested straight from the anus without chewing.

Diarrhoea and caecotroph accumulation
- Many cases of apparent 'diarrhoea' in the rabbit are in fact due to inadequate caecotroph ingestion relative to production
- The accumulation of soft uneaten caecotrophs around the anus mimics diarrhoea

Caecotroph accumulation
- Caecotrophs are usually produced only once or twice daily
- Soft but not liquid
- Covered in thin layer of mucus only
- Interspersed with normal hard dry pellets

ORGAN SYSTEMS

- Rabbits are usually otherwise well in themselves with good appetite
- On microscopy, caecotrophs contain large numbers of bacteria

Diarrhoea
- Produced throughout the day and night
- Not usually any normal pellets present
- May be associated with blood or excessive mucus
- On microscopy contains long fibre particles
- May be liquid
- May be foul smelling
- As caecotrophy develops between 3 and 6 weeks, under this age diarrhoea is more likely

True diarrhoea, due to the subsequent alterations in fluid and electrolyte balance, and disturbance of GI flora and motility, is a life threatening condition.
- Caecotroph accumulation is covered on p. 13.

Mucoid enteropathies
- Mucus production can be seen associated with diarrhoea, with passage of normal faeces, and with lack of faecal output
- A number of similar syndromes exist where mucus production occurs
- These syndromes occur most commonly around the time of weaning, when the caecal microflora is becoming established

'Mucoid enteritis'
- A general term used by rabbit fanciers to include any condition where there is mucoid diarrhoea or faeces with excessive mucoid coating, rather than watery scours
- As this most commonly occurs around weaning, other GI conditions (especially coccidiosis and antibiotic associated diarrhoeas) have become grouped into this classification, and mucoid enteritis should not be regarded as a single disease entity

Mucoid enteropathy
- Described by Okerman in 1994
- It is termed enteropathy rather than enteritis because inflammation is not a marked character of the disease
- Outbreaks occur, although other disease entities may be to blame. Post-weaning rabbits, undergoing the additional stress of removal from their mothers, are mainly affected, although adults, especially the mothers of affected litters, are sometimes affected
- Individual adults on a poor diet and subjected to stress, may also present with mucoid enteropathy. In addition to the general clinical signs of these disease syndromes, there is lethargy, a 'glazed' facial expression, anorexia and either an absence of faecal production, or clear mucus only
- Abdominal pain, evidenced by tooth grinding, a hunched posture and reluctance to move, is a feature; PU/PD is often a feature

Cause
- Unknown, although histological evidence is suggestive of a dysautonomia, resulting in a functional gut obstruction through lack of neuronal control of the colon
  o Faster growing rabbits are worst affected, suggesting that high dietary protein and carbohydrate intakes may have some effect on susceptibility and/or progression
  o A low fibre diet also predisposes rabbits to this condition
- Loss of peristaltic movement leads to a build-up of clear mucus within the colon
- The caecum becomes impacted, and often the caecum and proximal colon fill with a hard dry mass of ingesta
- Fluid build-up in the stomach and small intestine leads to a 'hot water-bottle' feel and sound to the abdomen

ORGAN SYSTEMS

- Aspiration pneumonia (due to stomach content overflow or dysphagia) is a finding in approximately 60% of animals at post-mortem examination
- Secondary enterotoxaemia is also seen
- Mortality reaches 60–100% in young rabbits

Rabbit epizootic enterocolitis/rabbit enzootic mucoid enteropathy
- First appeared in France in 1996
- This syndrome shows much in common with mucoid enteropathy, and may be the same condition, but information spread has been limited by the lack of published English language research
- A recent survey of commercial rabbit breeders (Jones & Duff, 2001) revealed that 14/17 commercial breeders had suffered losses of rabbits showing suggestive signs

Clinical history and signs
- Usually affects animals at the time of weaning, up to 7 weeks
- Mortality of up to 70% seen
- Abdominal enlargement due to huge distension of colon with mucus
- Epidemiological analysis of the 'outbreaks' suggest a viral cause, although histopathology has not consistently demonstrated this

Treatment
- Control of secondary infections with
  ○ Antibiotics
  ○ Probiotics/transfaunation
- GI prokinetics
- Supportive fluids and nutrition
- Analgesia

Prevention of mucoid enteropathies
- Correct diet
- Avoidance and reduction of stress at weaning and moving on
- Probiotic use

- Prophylactic antibiotics should be avoided
- Good hygiene
- Biosecurity measures to avoid potential viral infection

Incorrect diet
- Incorrect diet alone may cause either diarrhoea or caecotroph accumulation
  ○ This is often transient, typically following the addition of large amounts of unfamiliar foodstuffs (e.g. lettuce), and self limiting as long as the rabbit is not losing fluid, and is still eating and drinking, and is not systemically unwell
- Some cases, e.g. following feeding items (such as grass clippings) that precipitate a change in caecal flora, are more serious, and are covered under Caecal dysbiosis/enterotoxaemia, p. 140
- In some cases, food can move through the stomach too rapidly or in too dense a matrix for acid neutralization of bacteria to take place
- This can lead to intestinal dysbiosis
- Most cases of dietary induced chronic 'diarrhoea' are in fact caecotroph accumulation
- Those that are not usually respond to the same dietary changes as does caecotroph accumulation (i.e. higher fibre, lower carbohydrate, fat and protein)
- A change to a hay only diet (if the rabbit will accept it) as an exclusion diet, and the slow reintroduction of one vegetable type at a time once GI symptoms have cleared, is advised
- Probiotic use may be a useful adjunct treatment

Neonatal colibacillosis
- *Escherichia coli* related diarrhoea at 1–14 days
- Rabbit-EPEC: similar strain to the enteropathogenic strains isolated from human infants

- Adhesion factors allow attachment to the microvillus border: attaching and effacing *E. coli*
- *E. coli* is not a normal isolate from the rabbit at this age
- Indiscriminate use of antibiotics, poor hygiene and stress are predisposing factors

Clinical signs

- Watery diarrhoea
- Stomach full of undigested milk on post-mortem examination
- Abdomen stained inside and out by diarrhoea on examination or post-mortem examination

Diagnosis

- Clinical signs
- Isolation of *Escherichia coli* from faeces or intestinal contents

Treatment

- Antibiotics (based on culture and sensitivity)
- Supportive care
- Prognosis poor: mortality approaches 100%

Post-weaning colibacillosis

- *Escherichia coli* infection in post-weaning rabbits is less common due to acidic gastric pH
- *E. coli* may be found in the normal adult rabbit in cases of dysbiosis for other reasons, so isolation of *E. coli* is not, in itself, diagnostic
- Indiscriminate use of antibiotics, poor hygiene and stress are predisposing factors

Clinical signs

- Watery, light brown or red, foul smelling diarrhoea
- Intussusception and rectal prolapse may occur
- Longitudinal 'paintbrush' haemorrhages on caecal wall at post-mortem examination

Diagnosis

- Culture of heavy growths of *Escherichia coli and* gross or histopathological evidence.

Cryptosporidium parvum

- Can cause transitory diarrhoea in unweaned rabbits
- Unlikely to be significant in adult rabbits
- Self-limiting but slows growth markedly
- Organisms can be detected on ileal or jejunal smears or histopathology
- An ELISA test exists
- *NB: Zoonotic* in immune suppressed humans

Flagellates

- A number of different protozoa species are found in rabbit intestinal contents and occasionally faeces, e.g.
  - *Giardia duodenalis*
  - *Monocercomonas cuniculi*
  - *Retortamonas cuniculi*
  - *Isotricha*-like species
  - *Entamoeba cuniculi*
- More commonly found in faeces of rabbits with diarrhoea
- Presence is normal
- Increased numbers in faeces are a product, rather than a cause of, the diarrhoea
- Catarrhal enteritis due to *Giardia duodenalis* reported

Yeasts

- The presence of yeasts (*Cyniclomyces* (syn *Saccharomyces*) *guttulatulus*) in faeces and caecal contents is normal
- Increased numbers in diarrhoea states are a consequence of altered caecal control rather than suggestive of a pathological organism

Salmonella

- *Salmonella typhimurium* or *S. enteriditis* infections can occur, but are uncommon
- Diarrhoea is not always a feature

Other clinical signs
- Septicaemia, pyrexia, depression, abortion, metritis and death

Diagnosis at post-mortem examination
- Petechiation and congestion of multiple organs
- Necrotic foci on liver and spleen
- Culture from affected organs or faeces

Treatment
- Antibiotics based on culture and sensitivity may be attempted, but the *zoonotic* implications often necessitate euthanasia

Tyzzer's disease
- *Clostridium piliforme* (previously *Bacillus piliformis*) is a motile, spore forming, obligate intracellular bacterium
- Affects caecum, intestine and liver
- Uncommon in pet rabbits
- Disease often occurs following stress factors

Clinical signs
- Watery diarrhoea
- Depression
- Death
- Usually acute disease in young rabbits, with older individuals developing a more chronic disease with weight loss, intermittent diarrhoea and ill-thrift

Diagnosis at post-mortem examination
- Oedematous intestinal wall
- Necrotic foci in colonic mucosa and liver
- Myocardial lesions may be present

Treatment
- Palliative or preventative
- Intracellular nature of organism limits the effectiveness of antibiotics once infection has taken hold

Prevention
- Bacterial spores are killed by 0.3% sodium hypochlorite

Tularaemia
- *Francisella tularensis*
- Uncommon cause of enteritis and typhlitis

Other bacteria
- *Pseudomonas* and *Campylobacter* spp. have been reported to cause diarrhoea
- Prevention by good hygiene, especially with shared water drinking systems
- Treatment with appropriate antibiotics

Coronavirus
- Present in normal healthy adult rabbits
- Causes diarrhoea in 3–10 week old rabbits
- High morbidity (50%)
- Most affected animals die within 24 hours

Clinical signs
- Lethargy, diarrhoea, abdominal swelling

Diagnosis at post-mortem examination
- Fluid caecal contents
- Intestinal villous atrophy on histopathology

Rotavirus
- Uncommon in individual adult pet rabbits
- More common in groups of younger rabbits
- Rotaviral infection alone is mild and self-limiting
- Most animals are unaffected; some develop mild diarrhoea
- In conjunction with bacterial pathogens or opportunists, more serious

Clinical signs
- Mortality approaches 80% in rabbits aged 30–80 days
- Severe anorexia
- Greenish-yellow watery diarrhoea
- Dehydration

Diagnosis at post-mortem examination
- Ileum most affected
- Lymphocytic infiltration of lamina propria

ORGAN SYSTEMS

- Villous atrophy with swelling, rounding and desquamation of enterocytes

Intestinal coccidiosis

- There are 11 species of intestinal coccidia
- Vary greatly in their pathogenicity, and the site of their pathologic effect
- The most commonly identified species in clinical disease are *Eimeria perforans*, *E. magna*, *E. media* and *E. irresidua*
- Clinical infections can occur at any age, but are most common in young, growing rabbits, partly because one of the most important clinical signs (stunted growth) is only evident at this age
- Clinical signs can occur before oocysts are evident in the faeces

Other clinical signs

- Mild intermittent diarrhoea, with or without mucus or blood
- Weight loss
- Dehydration
- Secondary bacterial infections
- Intussusception
- Rectal prolapse
- Death

Post-mortem findings

- Inflammation, ulceration and haemorrhage of intestinal epithelium
- Site of lesions dependent on species involved

Definitive diagnosis

- Difficult, as clinical signs are similar to those of colibacillosis and other enteric diseases
- Also, coccidia are often present alongside other infections as a subclinical infestation
- Demonstration of high numbers of oocysts in faeces or intestinal contents, or confirmation of moderately high numbers of a recognized pathogenic species, ideally in conjunction with lesions in sites typical of that species, are required for definitive diagnosis

Treatment

- Drugs that are effective against intestinal coccidia include:
  - Robenidine
  - Sulpha drugs
  - Clopidol
  - Amprolium
- Sulpha drugs have the advantage of providing some effect against secondary bacterial infections that may occur alongside coccidiosis

Prevention

- Oocysts require 2 days to sporulate in faeces
  - Hence, infective oocysts do not occur in caecotrophs
- Preventing access to faeces over 2 days old is therefore effective in avoiding a build-up of pathogenic numbers.
  - This can be achieved by the use of wire flooring (although this has strong negative welfare implications), deep litter systems (where heat and ammonia destroy the oocysts, though these systems are bad for respiratory health), or diligent hygiene.

Cessation or reduction of faecal production

(Ileus, caecal impaction/tympany, megacolon, etc.)

- The reduction of faecal production (complete cessation, reduction in either size of faecal pellet or numbers) may be due to stasis anywhere within the gut, from mouth to colon, and is usually accompanied by anorexia
- Gastric stasis is covered in Oesophageal disorders, p. 123, Gastric disorders, p. 124, and Gastrointestinal stasis, p. 31)
- The other main site of stasis is the caecum/colon
- Other symptoms include:
  - Weight loss
  - Abdominal enlargement

- ○ Abdominal pain
- ○ Decreased activity
- The reasons for this syndrome are described on p. 31

Foreign bodies
- Foreign bodies distal to the sacculus rotundus are rare
- Most foreign bodies of sufficient size to cause obstruction lodge at sites proximal to the caecum
- Clay-based cat litter can accumulate in the caecum
- Large numbers of *Passalurus ambiguus*, the rabbit pinworm, may occur in the caecal ampulla and colon, but are rarely associated with blockage
- Large solid lumps of caecal contents may move into the narrower colon, obstructing it

Extraluminal obstructions
- These can occur due to neoplasia, abscesses, adhesions or torsion (see Small intestinal disorders, p. 131)
- Recto-anal papillomas occur commonly, but whilst they are friable and bleed easily, they are rarely associated with significant problems

Hypomotility of the large intestine
Dysautonomia
- Similar to grass sickness in horses
- Other autonomic signs, e.g. mydriasis, reduced tear production and salivation, may be seen
- Diagnosed at histopathology

Megacolon
- Whilst the caecum is the usual site of impaction, megacolon, a condition where the colon is full of chronically accumulated faeces in large clumps, has been reported
- The cause of this condition is not known, but it may affect white rabbits with dark ears and spots disproportionately commonly

- This megacolon syndrome, described in homozygous spotted rabbits, results in caecal obstipation, but there is uncertainty as to whether this is a true dysautonomia

Non-specific hypomotility disorders
- Caecal motility is regulated by the fusus coli
- The fusus coli is very sensitive to circulating catecholamines, with the result that stress reduces gut motility

Potential causes
- Any source of pain, for example
  - ○ Dental pain, e.g. spurs on cheek teeth abrading the tongue
  - ○ Musculoskeletal pain, e.g. arthritis
  - ○ Foot pain, e.g. plantar pododermatitis
  - ○ Visceral pain, e.g. GI bloating
  - ○ Perineal pain, e.g. urine scalding +/− flystrike
  - ○ Urological pain, e.g. urolithiasis
- Predators, e.g. cats, dogs, foxes
- Dominance issues
  - ○ Bullying by another rabbit
  - ○ Hierarchical disputes
- Sudden diet changes
- Transportation
- Weather or temperature changes
- Loss of companion
- Unavailability of water or food
- Loud noises, e.g. fireworks, thunderstorms
- Change in routine, e.g. sudden day-length changes
- Obesity
- Chronic dehydration
- Toxins affecting GI motility, e.g. lead
- Neurological disorders, e.g. spinal damage
- Caecal dysbiosis/enterotoxaemia
- Impaction with, e.g. clay cat litter, bulk laxatives

Diagnosis
- Diagnosis is on clinical presentation

ORGAN SYSTEMS

ORGAN SYSTEMS

- A full history to investigate potential causal factors should be taken, with reference to the list of possible initiators given above
- Physical examination should consist of a full clinical examination, with special reference to oral examination and abdominal palpation, auscultation and percussion
- Radiography can be used to demonstrate gas accumulation, foreign bodies, clumped faeces in the colon, etc.

Treatment
- Caecal impaction carries a poor prognosis
- As for gastric stasis, treatment is a combination of addressing the underlying cause(s) and supportive therapy (primarily fluids, nutrition, analgesia and GI prokinetics)
- Liquid paraffin may be beneficial in softening the caecal contents
- Avoidance of NSAIDs which inhibit prostaglandins (e.g. ketoprofen) and thus may inhibit the fusus coli may be helpful
- Use of prostaglandins (e.g. dinoprost) to stimulate caecal motility has been suggested, but with little supporting data

Gastric stasis and anorexia
There is also an interrelationship with gastric motility in that the stomach possesses very little intrinsic motility, and is partly driven by caecocolonic contractions.

A reduction in ingesta throughput from the stomach, particularly if the more fibrous components are retained in the stomach, in turn means that the caecum is starved of suitable substrate to ferment and drive hindgut motility. Primary anorexia (starvation, dental disease, renal disease, etc.) can initiate this.

Inflammatory bowel disease
- Cowpat-like faeces
- Responds to salazopyrin or steroid therapy

Caecal dysbiosis/enterotoxaemia
Enterotoxaemia can occur as a result of disturbance to the normal caecal microbiological flora (dysbiosis).

Causative factors
- Changed caecal pH favouring clostridial growth (normal caecal pH 5.9–6.8)
- High fermentable carbohydrate diet leading to a more acidic environment
- Low fibre diet (decreased VFA production) leading to a more alkaline environment
- High protein diet (breakdown to ammonia) leading to a more alkaline environment
- Reduced gut motility (as a result of the above, or any other reason)
- Concurrent poor hygiene
- Stress
- Concurrent disease
- Antibiotic administration
  - Especially oral antibiotics, those with good diffusion characteristics, and particularly those selectively affecting Gram-positive bacteria and anaerobic bacteria, e.g. clindamycin, lincomycin, penicillins and cephalosporins, erythromycin, tylosin
  - These have a variable effect: oral lincomycin nearly always produces a severe immediate enterocolitis, whereas parenteral penicillins do not commonly produce ill effects, particularly if the rabbit's diet is appropriately high in fibre providing buffering effects on caecal pH
- Various clostridia occur normally in the rabbit GIT, or are not associated with endotoxaemia
  - *Clostridium spiroforme*, however, produces iota-like toxin and is highly pathogenic to rabbits
  - *C. difficile* or *C. perfringens* may also be involved to a lesser extent

- Enterotoxaemia occurs most commonly in the few weeks immediately after weaning, at which time the caecal pH is still stabilizing, but it can occur at any age
- In acute cases the rabbit becomes depressed, bloated and anorectic
  - Brown watery diarrhoea is passed, which may contain blood and/or mucus
  - The abdomen may have a 'hot water-bottle' feel and sound
  - As the disease progresses the animal becomes shocked and hypothermic, and death occurs within 24–48 hours
- In the cases of antibiotic related enterotoxaemia, death may not occur until up to 3 weeks after cessation of the antibiotic therapy, as these drugs may also suppress the *Clostridium*
- Chronic cases can be seen, with intermittent diarrhoea, anorexia and weight loss; such cases may also develop pseudomembranous colitis
- Diagnosis is based on history, clinical signs and radiographic findings of generalized gassy ileus (though be aware the normal rabbit caecum contains gas pockets), and supported by typical post-mortem findings of petechiae and ecchymosis of the serosal surface, and haemorrhage and mucus on the mucosa of the proximal colon, caecum and appendix
  - Definitive diagnosis is on identification of *C. spiroforme* spiral forms in faeces or intestinal contents

Treatment
- Aggressive supportive care
  - Fluids
  - Nutritional support, especially provision of long fibre
  - Warmth
- Analgesia

- GI prokinetics
- Probiotics
- Proprietary preparations or transfaunation with healthy rabbit caecotrophs
- Cholestyramine to absorb iota-like toxin
  - Effective in absorbing toxins produced in antibiotic (clindamycin) associated enterotoxaemia
- Vitamin C at 100 mg/kg daily (anti-iota toxin effect) may reduce toxin production and absorption
- Antibiotics
  - Vancomycin most effective, but in human medicine this is reserved for resistant staphylococcal enterotoxaemia, so its use is limited
  - Metronidazole may be useful in *C. spiroforme* infection
  - Many antibiotics with *in vitro* effectiveness appear useless in practice, e.g. chloramphenicol, sulphaquinoxaline
  - Cases that apparently respond to antibiotics may then relapse once the treatment is stopped.

Prevention
- Multivalent clostridial sheep vaccines have been suggested
- However, the reason that sheep vaccines are multivalent is that there is little cross protection between clostridial species, and hence commercial vaccines (which do not contain *C. spiroforme*) are unlikely to offer protection against this specific organism
- Toxoids produced from specific strains of *C. spiroforme* have been shown to be protective
- Otherwise, prevention is by provision of a high fibre diet and reduction of stress
- Probiotics may be useful

Haematochezia and melaena
(See Haematochezia and melaena, p. 35)

HEPATOBILIARY TRACT DISORDERS

DIAGNOSIS

History and clinical signs
See also Jaundice, p. 46 and Ascites, p. 8.
- Icterus
- Ascites
- Weight loss
- Stunted growth
- Anorexia
- Diarrhoea
- Collapse
- Neurological signs
- Abdominal enlargement
- Hepatomegaly

Laboratory tests for liver disease
- Fungal culture of mouldy food or bedding
  - Examination for *Aspergillus* spp. giving rise to aflatoxicosis
- Haematology
  - Full haematology should be performed
  - Anaemia is expected in any chronic disease process
  - Regenerative vs. non-regenerative
  - Regenerative may indicate haemolytic process
  - Non-regenerative may indicate chronic inflammation
  - White blood cell changes are very variable, and depend on the exact nature of the disease
  - Heterophilia in presence of infection
  - Heteropaenia with sepsis
  - Leucopaenia in presence of severe infection
  - Monocytosis may indicate chronic infection
- Biochemistry
  - See Liver enzymes and associated parameters, p. 79
- Faecal analysis
  - Hepatic coccidia (*Eimeria stiedai*)
    — Significant finding if oocysts found in faeces or intestinal contents

- Liver fluke
  - — *Fasciola hepatica* eggs in faeces significant
- Urinalysis
  - Bilirubin and urobilinogen on dipsticks are not reliable tests
- Other clinical pathology
  - Histopathology or cytology from liver biopsies or impression smears
  - Microscopy on samples of bile or intestinal contents for *E. stiedai* oocysts or *F. hepatica* eggs.

Diagnostic imaging of the liver
Radiography
- On the lateral view the liver is visible within the ribcage caudal to the diaphragm and with a small triangle projecting caudal and slightly ventral to the xiphisternum
- The stomach sits dorsal to this

Ultrasonography
- Similar to feline
- Minimal fur should be clipped, and care should be taken not to wet the animal excessively, to avoid chilling the rabbit, especially smaller individuals
- Gel can be warmed, both to avoid hypothermia and to be more comfortable to the conscious animal
- The liver can usually be viewed via the ventral abdomen
- Ultrasound provides useful information about internal liver architecture, but is complicated by the presence of large amounts of gas within the intestines
  - Also provides good visualization of biliary tree, including bile stasis, and liver fluke adults within the bile duct
- Hepatic lipidosis
  - Generalized increased echogenicity
- Focal changes, e.g. abscessation, neoplasia
  - Normal liver should be homogeneous
  - Localized areas of varied echogenicity

- Abscess is variably hypoechoic to hyperechoic or mixed, with hyperechoic capsule
- Neoplasia is hyperechoic

Liver biopsy

- Definitive diagnosis of liver disease requires histopathological examination
- Can be carried out either percutaneously (ideally with ultrasound guidance to avoid and identify iatrogenic injury and target lesions) or via exploratory laparotomy or laparoscopy
  - Either option should be carried out under GA
- Percutaneous biopsy most useful in generalized disease processes, e.g. hepatic lipidosis
- Biopsy at exploratory laparoscopy/laparotomy permits more precise biopsy of focal lesions, although ultrasound guidance in experienced hands may allow accurate localization of internal hepatic lesions

Fine needle aspirate

- Only really useful in very diffuse conditions, e.g. hepatic lipidosis
- Safer in terms of being less likely to create serious haemorrhage or damaging abscess capsule, allowing purulent material into abdomen

Tru-cut biopsy

- Harvests a larger sample
- Relatively more representative than a fine needle aspirate
- Still risks missing focal lesions
- Increased risk of haemorrhage or rupture of abscess

Laparoscopy

- Requires a relatively small incision
- Reduces surgical time and leads to a more rapid recovery
- Appropriate biopsy forceps allow precise sampling of specific areas

- Concurrent ultrasonography to identify internal lesions is possible
- Good quality equipment is expensive
- Significant operator skill is required to achieve good quality biopsy in a similar time to that of the average surgeon performing a laparotomy
- Haemorrhage is less easy to control
- Larger biopsies or liver lobectomies cannot be carried out
- Avoidance of large gas filled intestines can be difficult without traumatizing them

Laparotomy

- Allows good visualization of liver and other organs
- Allows for sample of any size to be taken
- Allows lesions to be identified and sampled accurately
- Surgical excision of lesions or entire lobe possible
- Does not require specialized skills
- Larger incision required
- Longer anaesthetic time than skilled laparoscopy
- Recovery slower, and more risk of wound breakdown, self trauma, etc.

CAUSES OF LIVER DISEASE

Trauma

- Abdominal trauma, e.g. road traffic collision, fall, predation, crushing or kick injuries
- Caudate lobe torsion
  - Relatively mobile caudate lobe may undergo torsion
  - Differential for sudden death or acute abdomen

Hepatic coccidiosis

- *Eimeria stiedai* infection
  - Must be distinguished from nonpathogenic species of intestinal coccidiosis

- Causes anything from decreased weight gain of young, to ascites, icterus, diarrhoea, anorexia and death
- Inhabits bile duct epithelia and causes biliary obstruction with time
  - Abscess-like lesions exude cloudy bile when incised

Diagnostic tests
- Hepatomegaly on radiography
- Raised ALKP, ALT, AST, GGT, LDH and total bilirubin
- Enlarged gall bladder on ultrasonography

Definitive diagnosis
- Clinical signs of hepatic disease *and* E. stiedai oocysts

Treatment
- Control of organism with sulpha drugs, clopidol, toltrazuril or amprolium until immunity develops
- Removing access to faeces over 2 days old prevents ingestion of viable sporulated oocysts
  - This can be by use of mesh floors, deep pit systems where heat destroys the oocysts, or ideally by diligent cleaning

Hepatic lipidosis
- The end stage result of prolonged anorexia, particularly in obese animals and pregnant does
  - Anorexia results in fat stores being mobilized for energy
  - Only minor stress is needed in obese rabbits to induce free fatty acid mobilization
  - Hepatocytes can become full of lipid and develop necrosis
  - Typical signs include anorexia, depression, convulsions, abortion and death

Diagnostic tests
- Hepatomegaly on radiography
- Hypoechoic appearance on ultrasonography

- Ketonuria
- Elevated blood ketones
- Elevated bile acids
- Lipaemia, elevated cholesterol and triglycerides

Definitive diagnosis
- Hepatic biopsy and histopathology

Treatment
- Supportive treatment concentrating on provision of glucose for metabolism; IV or IO glucose-containing fluids and aggressive supportive nutrition
- Treatment of the underlying cause, which may include termination of pregnancy if the rabbit is a surgical candidate
- Prognosis is very poor, and worsens as the disease process continues

Hepatic neoplasia
- Primary hepatic neoplasms reported include bile duct adenoma and carcinomas
- Hepatic coccidiosis and other chronic irritants may be initiating factors
- Multifocal neoplasms include lymphosarcoma
- The most common metastatic neoplasm of rabbits is uterine adenocarcinoma

Diagnostic tests
- Radiography may reveal hepatomegaly
- Ultrasound examination may show hypoechoic lesions
- Elevated levels of liver enzymes
- Hepatic necrosis: ALT, AST, LDH, bile acids, total bilirubin
- Bile stasis due to biliary tree obstruction: ALKP, ALT, AST, GGT, LDH, bile acids, total bilirubin

Definitive diagnosis
- Biopsy and histopathology

Treatment
- As with canine and feline hepatic neoplasia
  - Lymphoma may be approached with similar chemotherapy protocols, although remission is extremely unlikely
- Surgery is unlikely to be curative except in the case of very discrete primary neoplasms with no further metastasis
  - Most hepatic neoplasms have miliary metastasis, and carry a very poor prognosis

Toxic liver damage
Causes
- Iatrogenic toxicity with drugs such as NSAIDs
- Heavy metal toxicity, e.g. lead
- Plant toxins, e.g. avocado, *Crotalaria* spp.
- Fungal toxins, e.g. *Aspergillus* aflatoxins (particularly aflatoxin B_1)
- Pine and cedar wood shavings as bedding or litter tray substrate

Signs
- Anorexia, depression
- Weight loss
- Neurological signs
- Icterus

History
- A thorough history, including exposure to plant species indoors and out and type of bedding material, is necessary
- Extremely high lipid intakes (usually only seen with parenteral lipid administration) can lead to liver pathology

Diagnostic tests
- Raised serum enzymes suggestive of hepatocellular damage:
  - ALT, AST, LDH, bile acids, total bilirubin
- Testing food for aflatoxins

Diagnosis
- On clinical signs, history of eating affected material (sample of known toxic plant, mouldy hay which grows *Aspergillus* spp. on fungal media), recent access to pine or cedar shavings, or specific toxin test, e.g. blood lead analysis

Treatment
- Specific antidotes if possible, e.g. sodium calcium EDTA for lead poisoning
- Inducing vomiting not possible
- Gastric lavage or administration of GI absorbants may be appropriate in early cases
- Removal of inappropriate bedding

Abscessation
- The liver is a possible site of abscess formation, either via haematogenous (portal or systemic) spread from other foci of infection, trauma, or extension of other abscesses within the abdominal cavity

Diagnostic tests
- As for neoplasia, raised liver enzymes suggestive of either hepatocellular damage, or bile stasis, depending on the exact site of the abscess
- Haematology may reveal, as with any abscess, either no changes whatsoever in the white blood cell count, heterophilia and lymphopaenia with no total white blood cell count increase, or an increase, due mainly to heterophils
- Radiography may reveal focal hepatomegaly
- Ultrasound examination may reveal hepatomegaly and focal hyperechoic changes.

Definitive diagnosis
- Visual confirmation of abscess at laparotomy or laparoscopy, and/or aspiration of purulent material

ORGAN SYSTEMS

Treatment

- Medical treatment alone is likely to be unrewarding, due to the thick nature of rabbit pus and the surrounding abscess capsule
- Total surgical excision, if possible, is curative, although other abscesses may be present, there may be widespread bacterial infection (e.g. *Pasteurella multocida*), and there may be other immune suppressive problems (e.g. dental disease) that may also need addressing

Tyzzer's disease

- Uncommon in pet rabbits
- *Clostridium piliforme* (previously *Bacillus piliformis*)
  - Gram-negative organism, which is an obligate intracellular parasite, transmitted faeco-orally and able to form spores which are difficult to eliminate
  - Causes disease ranging from ill-thrift to anorexia, diarrhoea, depression, dehydration and death
  - Chronic weight loss may occur in older animals

Diagnostic tests

- Raised liver enzymes suggestive of hepatocellular damage, e.g. ALT, AST, LDH, bile acids, total bilirubin
- Multiple necrotic foci on visualization of the liver

Definitive diagnosis

- Identification of the organism on culture is difficult, and generally diagnosis is at post mortem, on gross and histopathological appearance

Treatment

- In groups, oxytetracycline has been suggested early in an outbreak, although culling and restocking is often carried out to eliminate the infection
- In individual animals, supportive therapy (fluids, nutrition, antibiotics, e.g. tetra-cyclines) may be successful, but long term intestinal damage is likely
- Prevention is by minimizing stress, quarantining new arrivals and good hygiene, including disinfection with 0.3% sodium hypochlorite to eliminate spores

Liver fluke (*Fasciola hepatica*)

- Usually only infects rabbits that graze wet pasture (river and pond edges) inhabited by the water snails that act as the intermediate host
  - Signs include cachexia, lethargy, ascites and death

Diagnostic tests

- Liver parameters may be elevated, especially those affected by bile stasis due to biliary tree obstruction, e.g. ALKP, ALT, AST, GGT, LDH, bile acids, total bilirubin
- Gall bladder enlargement, and even adult flukes, may be identified on ultrasound examination

Definitive diagnosis

- Identification of fluke eggs in the faeces or adult parasites in the bile duct on laparoscopy/laparotomy/post-mortem examination

Treatment

- Single dose of praziquantel at 5–10 mg/kg

Prevention

- Avoidance of grazing in wetland areas

Taenia spp. tapeworm cysts

- Whilst intestinal cestode infestations are extremely rare in domestic rabbits, cysticercosis with *Taenia pisiformis* and *T. serialis* are much more common
- 'Cysts' form on the abdominal surfaces, and to a lesser extent, the liver
  - These are usually incidental findings
  - Tapeworm migration through the liver can cause necrotic and fibrous lesions

Diagnosis

- Liver enzymes may be raised if there is bile duct stasis or significant hepatocellular damage
- Cysts may be observed on ultrasound or radiographic examination, or at laparotomy, often as an incidental finding

Treatment

- Drainage, with or without systemic or intralesional praziquantel administration, appears curative

Toxoplasmosis and E. cuniculi

- Have been reported to cause focal interstitial granulomatous hepatitis
  - Not believed to be a significant cause of liver disease

Viral haemorrhagic disease

- Most cases of rabbit VHD, or rabbit calicivirus, are acute to hyperacute, with death often occurring before any clinical signs are evident
- In those cases where clinical signs are present, these can include lethargy, depression, pyrexia, anorexia, tachypnoea, tachycardia, cyanosis, abdominal enlargement, diarrhoea, collapse, neurological signs including convulsions, and death
  - Haemorrhage from any or all body orifices may occur

Diagnosis

- Usually at post-mortem examination; hepatic portal necrosis is evident on histopathological examination
- IFA testing, electron microscopy or PCR/ELISA can be used to confirm infection

Treatment

- No treatment available
- Prevention is by vaccination and avoidance of infective animals or fomites (these can include shoes or pets that have covered ground infected by wild rabbits)

Bacterial and other infections from intestine via portal vein

(See also Section 4, p. 175)

- Colibacillosis
- Salmonellosis
  - May see pyrexia and diarrhoea
- Listeriosis
- Tularaemia
  - Zoonotic
  - Resilient non-spore forming obligate aerobe
  - Rare
  - Causes focal nodules and necrosis of liver and spleen
  - More severe infection in young animals
  - Isolation of organism difficult
  - Diagnosis usually at post mortem on histopathology
- Pseudotuberculosis (yersiniosis)
  - Nodular swelling and caseous necrosis seen
- Tuberculosis
- Toxoplasmosis
- Cryptosporidiosis
  - ELISA or faecal microscopy
  - These are all possible infective agents, spread from intestinal infection to the liver
  - They can be associated with both intestinal and hepatic disease at the same time, so clinical signs are many, but may include diarrhoea, anorexia, depression, lethargy, collapse, dehydration, ascites, icterus and death

Diagnostic tests

- Raised serum liver enzymes associated with either bile stasis or hepatic cellular necrosis
- Hepatomegaly on radiography or ultrasound examination

Diagnosis

- Identification of the causal organism in faeces, intestinal contents, or ideally from liver, together with suspicious clinical signs

ORGAN SYSTEMS

ORGAN SYSTEMS

Treatment
- In severe cases unrewarding, but early intervention with appropriate antibiotics (decided upon on the basis of culture and sensitivity) may be effective against susceptible organisms.
- Diseases such as yersiniosis can be extremely difficult, if not impossible, to eradicate. In colony situations this may necessitate culling and restocking, and even in individual cases its zoonotic potential *must* be taken into account when deciding on treatment options.

GENERAL SUPPORTIVE TREATMENT IN LIVER DISEASE

- A good quality, well balanced diet, possibly with supplementation of water-soluble vitamins which may be lacking due to impaired hepatic metabolism
- Milk thistle (*Silybum marianum*) (active ingredient, silymarin) has been suggested as an aid to hepatic regeneration, and may be given as the fresh plant or extract

SPLENIC AND PANCREATIC DISORDERS

SPLEEN

The rabbit spleen is flattened and elongated. It is attached to the dorsolateral surface of the greater curvature of the stomach. The normal spleen cannot be seen on radiography. It is smaller than in most animals, as gut associated lymphoid tissue accounts for 50% of total lymphoid tissue mass.

Splenomegaly
Causes
- VHD
- Toxoplasmosis
  - Acute toxoplasmosis leads to splenomegaly
  - Anorexia, lethargy, pyrexia, muscle tremors and weakness, and paresis may also be seen
- Salmonellosis
  - In acute *Salmonella* infection, the spleen may enlarge to ten times the normal size
  - Metritis may also occur in intact females; identification of the characteristic necrotic foci on the spleen and liver is at post mortem or upon laparotomy/laparoscopy
- Pseudotuberculosis (*Yersinia pseudotuberculosis*)

  - Uncommon in rabbits
  - Caseous necrosis of spleen may be seen at post mortem or upon laparotomy/laparoscopy
- Lymphosarcoma
- Tularaemia
  - Zoonotic
  - Resilient non-spore forming obligate aerobe
  - Rare
  - Causes focal nodules and necrosis of liver and spleen
  - More severe infection in young animals

PANCREAS

- The pancreas is a small, diffuse organ in the rabbit
- It is positioned between the transverse colon, stomach and duodenum, often surrounded in fat and difficult to find
- The pancreatic duct is separate from the bile duct in the rabbit, entering at the end of the duodenum
- Elevated amylase concentrations are seen in pancreatitis, pancreatic duct obstruction, and any abdominal insult indirectly affecting the pancreas

- Lipase is thought to rise following pancreatic cell damage, as with other species
- The pancreas does not have as important a role in glucose metabolism in the rabbit as in other species

DIABETES MELLITUS

Diabetes mellitus is the most commonly diagnosed endocrinopathy of rabbits. Its exact incidence is controversial, as it may commonly be misdiagnosed due to stress related hyperglycaemia and/or glycosuria. Insulin plays a relatively minor role in rabbits' glucose metabolism, with rabbits surviving long periods of time after experimental pancreatectomy.

A syndrome in NZW rabbits analogous to spontaneous human insulin dependent diabetes has been reported. Obesity does not seem to be a risk factor in this disease process.

Aetiology/risk factors
- NZW breed
- Obesity (in non-NZW rabbits)

Diagnosis
Glucose testing
Single elevated blood glucose readings, or glycosuria, are not diagnostic, especially when these samples have been taken in the stressful surroundings of the surgery. Differentials for these findings include:
- Hepatic lipidosis
- Starvation
- Stress
- Shock
- Halothane anaesthesia
- Hyperthermia
- Blood loss
- Early mucoid enteropathy
- Enteritis
- Glucose containing parenteral fluids recently administered
- Renal insufficiency
- Drug therapy, especially glucocorticoids

Repeatedly elevated blood glucose and glycosuria at home (using pocket glucometers on blood from spring loaded human glucose testing lancets, and test dipsticks, respectively) increase the index of suspicion for DM, although renal insufficiency and hepatic lipidosis remain differentials.

Other laboratory parameters
- The presence of ketonuria as well may raise the index of suspicion, but is more commonly seen with hepatic lipidosis
- Fructosamine has been explored as a diagnostic test and appears to correlate more accurately with clinical signs than glucose alone: this protein reflects the presence of hyperglycaemia over the previous 2–4 weeks
- Mild cases (that are not likely to require insulin) may be detected using an intravenous glucose tolerance test
- Increased serum ketones, cholesterol and triglycerides, and reduced serum potassium may also be seen

History and physical examination
- Polyuria: due to osmotic diuresis
- Polydipsia: secondary to polyuria
- Weight loss
- Polyphagia

Management
- Most cases can be controlled by normalizing the diet (see Nutritional requirements of rabbits, p. 105) and treating obesity in overweight individuals
- Oral hypoglycaemics and insulin are rarely indicated

ORGAN SYSTEMS

URINARY TRACT DISEASE

DIAGNOSIS OF RENAL DISORDERS

Renal failure:
- Given the functional reserve, a loss of 50–70% of renal function is required before renal parameters change and clinical signs develop

Azotaemia:
- An increase in urea and/or creatinine

Pre-renal:
- Reduced renal perfusion

Renal (primary):
- Primary renal disease

Post-renal:
- Obstruction or rupture of the urinary tract distal to the kidney

Uraemia:
- Clinical signs that develop as a result of raised urea and/or creatinine

History and clinical signs of renal insufficiency
- Polyuria
- Polydipsia
- Weight loss
- Inappetance
- Lethargy

Physical examination
- Abdominal palpation
  - Noting size, shape, texture of kidneys
  - Fullness of bladder
  - Site of any pain
- Mucous membrane colour and capillary refill time
- State of hydration
- Ophthalmic examination
- Uraemic ulceration of oral mucous membranes

Laboratory tests for renal disease
Urine sampling
- See Urinalysis, p. 83

- Provides useful information, especially in conjunction with blood work
- More sensitive indicator of early renal failure
- Sampling method must be taken into consideration when analysing results

Urine soaked bedding
- Whilst essentially useless for many parameters, soaked bedding that is stained red, giving a suspicion of haematuria, may be added to water, shaken, and sampled with a dipstick for haemoglobin
- Dietary pigments may also be differentiated from blood by their tendency to fluoresce under UV illumination

Free catch
- Free catch samples are difficult to obtain without contamination
  - Even using clean litter trays with non-absorbent litter, faeces is commonly voided at the same time
- Observation of micturition can be informative
  - The initial stage of urination allows free flow of urine from the bladder
  - The final phase involves abdominal contraction to expel the remaining urine from the bladder and cranial vagina
  - Any blood that has pooled in the latter from the uterus therefore tends to be passed in this stage
  - Increased straining during urination can be indicative of urolithiasis or 'sludge'
- Frequent small amounts of urine can be behavioural territory marking, but can also be a sign of decreased effective bladder volume due to 'sludge' build-up

Bladder expression
- Many rabbits will allow expression of the bladder whilst conscious

- Firm, gentle, continuous pressure is applied until urine begins to flow, and often the rest of the urine is expelled as normal

Cystocentesis

- Performed in a normal standing position with the hindlimbs raised to allow access to the ventral midline, or with the rabbit raised to stand vertically on its hindlimbs, or in dorsal recumbency
  - The bladder, when full, is large and often very flaccid, lying on the ventral abdominal floor cranial to the pelvic brim
  - Unless the bladder is full, easily palpated, and fixed in position, cystocentesis should not be performed due to the risk of caecum puncture

Catheterization

- Urethral catheterization is possible in both male and female rabbits, but may require sedation or anaesthesia
  - A 9F catheter is suitable for average sized rabbits of either sex
- Males are restrained in dorsal recumbency and the catheter advanced 1.5–4 cm into the urethra to obtain a sample
- The urethral orifice of the female is best accessed by passing the catheter along the ventral floor of the vagina with the doe in ventral recumbency
- Comparison of urine obtained by different methods may differentiate source of bleeding

Urinalysis

Appearance

- Rabbit urine can normally be anywhere from light yellow to dark brown, with varying amounts of suspended calcium, crystals and plant pigments
  - Cloudiness is rarely due to pyuria
  - Clear urine, unless the rabbit has a very low calcium intake, or is utilizing calcium heavily (growth, lactation, pregnancy), is abnormal

Timing of sampling

- The sample should be as fresh as possible, and in light of the amount of suspended particulate matter, crystalluria is of dubious significance in samples not examined shortly after collection
- Urine that has been stored in the bladder for a long time will be more concentrated, and will have the maximum yield of cellular material, blood, crystals, casts and glucose
- A more accurate urine pH will be obtained from a fresh sample
- The timing of obtaining this sample depends on the individual rabbit, but cannot always be guaranteed to be the morning

Testing methods

- Dipsticks are unreliable for anything other than blood/haemoglobin, pH, glucose and ketones
- Centrifugation and sampling of the sediment/supernatant interface may assist in obtaining useful samples for cytology, avoiding the presence of crystals in the sample
  - However, spinning can destroy fragile casts
  - Stains may be necessary for detection of *Encephalitozoon cuniculi*, e.g. trichrome
- Protein
  - Protein is more significant if found in very dilute urine
  - Urine protein loss may more accurately be assessed by urine protein/urine creatinine ratio
  - Values over unity are likely to indicate glomerular disease
- pH
  - Alkaline pH typical of herbivores (8–9)
  - Can drop to as low as 6 with catabolic states
  - Increases with age of sample due to bacterial metabolism

- Relative density (SG)
  - ○ Indicates ability to concentrate urine
  - ○ Ranges from 1.003 to 1.036
  - ○ Average 1.015
  - ○ Dipsticks particularly unreliable compared to refractometer measurements
  - ○ Urine SG is important to differentiate azotaemia into pre-renal and renal
    - — Pre-renal failure is usually associated with SG > 1.030 (increased)
    - — Primary renal failure associated with normal to under concentrated urine, <1.013
    - — Post-renal failure: urine can have varied SG
  - ○ Cannot be accurately interpretated following diuretics or rehydration.
- Calcium and crystalluria
  - ○ Degree of calciuria varies with calcium levels in the diet
  - ○ Calcium oxalate, calcium carbonate and ammonium magnesium carbonate (triple phosphate, struvite) crystals commonly occur and do not necessarily indicate urinary tract disease
  - ○ Urolithisasis is common
  - ○ Calculi may involve kidney, ureter, bladder or urethra
  - ○ Hydronephrosis and hydroureter may occur with upper urinary tract calculi
  - ○ Uroliths are radiodense due to their high mineral (calcium) content
- Leucocytes
  - ○ Indicative of inflammation in urogenital tract
  - ○ Only localize lesion to kidney (renal tubules) if casts are seen
- Casts
  - ○ Indicate renal pathology
  - ○ Deteriorate if sample is shaken, spun or stored too long
- Hyaline casts
  - ○ Protein
  - ○ Soluble at high pH, therefore rarely seen in rabbits
- Granular casts
  - ○ Cells, plasma proteins, lipids, etc.

- ○ Normal in small numbers
- ○ Large numbers normal following rehydration of previously dehydrated rabbit
- ○ Otherwise indicate nephrotoxic renal tubular injury or ischaemia
- ○ Deteriorate to waxy casts with time
- Renal epithelial casts
  - ○ Acute tubular necrosis
  - ○ Pyelonephritis
- Bacteria
  - ○ Primary bacterial urinary tract infections uncommonly symptomatic in rabbits
  - ○ Usually accompanied by WBC in urinary tract infections
- Biochemistry
  - ○ Creatinine more reliable than urea
  - ○ Ruptured bladders lead to urea and creatinine in the abdominal fluid
  - ○ Comparison of blood vs. fluid creatinine diagnostic
  - ○ Urea diffuses rapidly, therefore not diagnostic
- Blood
  - ○ Distinguish blood from haemoglobin/ myoglobin by dipstick or microscopy for RBCs
- Renal clearance testing
  - ○ Direct measurement of GFR requires measurement of clearance rates of substances excreted solely by the glomeruli
  - ○ These can be endogenous (creatinine) or exogenous (inulin)
  - ○ The latter is stressful and rarely justified; both techniques require the collection of urine over a 24-hour period, limiting their use

Blood parameters
Biochemistry
- See Azotaemia, p. 75

Haematology
- May see
  - ○ Non-regenerative anaemia
  - ○ Lymphopaenia

Table 3.3   Interpretation of changes seen on intravenous urography

Large smooth	⇒	Inflammatory, neoplastic or amyloid infiltrate, hydronephrosis, nephrolithiasis, renal cyst/abscess, hypertrophy, subcapsular urine or blood
Large irregular	⇒	Focal – tumour, abscess, cyst or haematoma; multifocal – cysts, lymphosarcoma
Normal size and shape	⇒	Normal, amyloid, glomerulonephritis or acute pyelonephritis
Normal size, irregular	⇒	Focal – infarct, inflammation, abscess or cyst; multifocal – polycystic or chronic pyelonephritis, multiple abscessation
Small smooth	⇒	Hypoplasia, amyloidosis or chronic glomerulonephritis
Small irregular	⇒	End stage, amyloidosis or infarct

From Sturgess (2003)

Imaging of the upper urinary tract

Survey radiography
- Soft tissue mineralization, especially dead or devitalised tissue
- Excessive mineralization of bones

Plain radiography
- To assess renal size and shape:
  - 1.25–1.75× the length of the second lumbar vertebra
  - Smooth regular outline
  - 'Kidney' shaped
- To check for presence of renal and ureteral calculi
- To check for signs of hydronephrosis and hydroureter

Intravenous urography
- 600–800 mg iodine/kg
  - Films taken at 0, 1, 5, 10, 15, 20 minutes
- Potential side effects include:
  - Acute renal failure (especially if already azotaemic)
  - Bradycardia/hypotension
  - Tachycardia/hypertension
  - Anaphylaxis

See Table 3.3 which details the interpretation of changes seen on intravenous urography.

Ultrasonography
- Sublumbar fat deposition common in the rabbit, especially older females
- Often impeded by air in GIT
- Renal cysts are usually clinically silent
- Dorsolateral flank approach avoids much of GIT
- Nephroliths may cast a shadow or reflection
- Hydronephrosis
  - Starting in the renal pelvis
  - Anechoic
- Hydroureter
  - Anechoic
  - Both of the above usually, but not always, due to nephrolithiasis or ureterolithiasis (hyperechoic)
- Focal changes
- Cysts
  - Anechoic
- Abscesses
  - Variable
  - From hypoechoic to hyperechoic depending on exact consistency of purulent material

○ Complex appearance within a hyper-echoic capsule possible
○ Calcification hyperechoic, with reflection or shadowing possible
• Haemorrhage
○ Anechoic, possibly with visible clots
• Ischaemia/infarcts
○ Hypoechoic, with calcification possible, as above

Renal biopsy
• Most useful in early renal failure
• Most useful for diffuse rather than focal lesions
• Indicated in unresponsive cases where kidney pathology identified
• Contraindicated where overt infection or hydronephrosis present
• Has been reported for definitive diagnosis of *Encephalitozoon cuniculi*
• Methodology as in the cat
• Complications include:
○ Haemorrhage, leading to:
— Urinary tract obstruction
— Infarction, thromboembolism and/or ischaemia
○ Aggravation of renal failure
○ Leakage of urine into abdomen

CAUSES OF RENAL DISEASE

Encephalitozoon cuniculi
• Mild/moderate proteinuria may be seen in affected rabbits
• Renal damage caused is usually mild and not usually of clinical significance
• *E. cuniculi* may be a factor in chronic renal failure
• May lead to renal fibrosis, obstructing urine flow
• Urinary incontinence with *E. cuniculi* is due to neurological impairment, not renal pathology
• Histopathological examination of kidney may reveal infection in rabbits where serology is negative

Interstitial nephritis
• Has been reported as a cause of soft tissue mineralization, and bony over-mineralization

Nephrolithiasis
• Formation of calculi, usually in the renal pelvis
○ High calcium and/or vitamin D intake
○ Reduced calcium excretion due to renal insufficiency
○ Calculi can accrete gradually to a large size
○ Renal pelvic dilatation and atrophy can result
○ Severe renal damage and insufficiency may have occurred by the time the condition is diagnosed
○ May be unilateral or (usually) bilateral, although commonly one kidney is affected far more seriously than the other
○ Surgical treatment options are well described, and include pyelolithotomy, nephrotomy or nephrectomy

Renal calcinosis
• A form of nephrolithiasis
• The entire renal parenchyma is affected, including the cortex
• A diffuse increase in radiodensity is seen throughout the kidney
• May be unilateral or bilateral
• Discrete renal pelvic uroliths are not necessarily seen with this condition
• Prognosis depends on the apparent function of the kidney(s) on IV excretory pyelogram and renal biochemistry

Neoplasia
• Renal carcinoma
• Embryonal nephroma
• Renal lymphosarcoma
○ Usually associated with multifocal organ involvement

Clinical signs
- Those of renal failure
- +/− urogenital tract bleeding
- And/or infection
- Some may be incidental findings at post mortem

Diagnosis
- Differentiation of kidney from other source of haemorrhage, pain, etc.
  - Ultrasound
  - IVU
  - Renal biopsy
- Survey radiographs should be taken to identify metastases.

Treatment
- Surgical resection if possible
- Nephrectomy has been reported
  - The main complication is the friable and well vascularized fat surrounding the kidney
  - The function of the other kidney should always be established before such surgery

Renal cysts
- Subcapsular cysts
- Familial renal cysts may be seen in some rabbits
- Multiple small cysts
- Autosomal recessive inherited trait (Lindsey & Fox, 1994)
- Often clinically insignificant, or totally asymptomatic
- May be palpated or identified by ultrasonography/IVU
- Differential diagnosis for hydronephrosis
- No treatment warranted

Renal agenesis
- Congenital absence of one kidney
- Autosomal recessive mutation in a colony of laboratory rabbits
- Has been reported in the Havana breed
- May be seen in both sexes

- In affected males there is often ipsilateral agenesis of the testis

Pyelonephritis, nephritis and renal abscesses
- Extension of urinary tract infection
  - Long term antimicrobial therapy required
  - Base antimicrobial choices on culture and sensitivity on cystocentesed urine
  - If culture negative, first choices include fluroquinolones, cephalosporins and potentiated sulphonamides
- Not common

Clinical signs
- Renal pain
- Renal enlargement
- Lethargy, depression, inappetance
- Pyrexia uncommon
- Hyperechoic renal pelvis on ultrasound examination
- Urine
  - Red and white cell casts
  - Pyuria
  - Bacteria on microscopy
  - Positive or negative culture

Laboratory changes
- Haematology and biochemistry
  - Anaemia
  - Heterophilia
  - Heteropaenia in sepsis
  - Lymphopaenia
  - Monocytosis in chronic infection

Ureteric disease
- Ureteral calculi
- Iatrogenic damage to ureter during speying
- Ectopic ureters

Clinical signs
- Abdominal/renal pain
- Inappetance
- Hunched stance
- Frequent attempts to urinate

Diagnosis
- Ultrasound of kidneys and ureters
- Plain radiographs to identify ureteral calculi
- IVU
- Surgical investigation

Treatment
- Surgery to relocate or deconstrict ureter, or remove calculus

ACUTE RENAL FAILURE

Rapid onset renal dysfunction leading to azotaemia.

Predisposing/initiating factors
- Pre-existing renal disease
- Pre-existing systemic disease
- Renal perfusion reduction
  - Shock
  - Hypovolaemia
  - Anaesthesia
  - Decreased cardiac output
- Hypothermia or heatstroke
- Sepsis, bacteraemia, pyrexia
- Fatty infiltration of the kidney in hepatic lipidosis
- Urinary tract infection
- Muscle damage, e.g. predator attacks
- Severe stress leading to reduction of renal blood flow
- Trauma to kidney
- Nephrotoxins
  - Therapeutics
    - Antibiotics especially aminoglycosides
    - EDTA, penicillamine, NSAIDs, IVU
    - Chemotherapy agents, e.g. cisplatin, cyclophosphamide, doxorubicin
    - Antifungals, e.g. amphotericin B
  - Non-therapeutics
    - Ethylene glycol, lead
  - Plant toxins, especially oxalates
    - Oak, aged dock leaves, beetroot leaves
  - Supplements
    - zinc, vitamin D overdose
- Severe GI disease or anorexia, leading to fluid and electrolyte imbalances
- Stress
  - Adrenaline markedly reduces renal blood flow
- Urinary obstruction
- Hypercalcaemia (dietary or pathological)

Diagnosis
History and clinical signs
- Polyuria
- Polydipsia
- Anuria/oliguria
- Perineal urine scalding
- Weight loss
- Inappetance
- Lethargy/depression
- Dehydration
- Uraemia
  - Halitosis, stomatitis, melaena
  - Depending on cause:
    - Renal pain
    - Renal enlargement
    - (Renal enlargement may be seen at post mortem due to congestive heart failure)
- History of drug administration, exposure to toxins, shock, predator attack
- Duration, severity and progression of clinical signs
  - But may indicate sudden deterioration of CRF

Urine production
- Anuria/oliguria
- Differentiate ARF from urinary tract obstruction
  - Latter will have enlarged bladder, hydronephrosis or hydroureter
- Cases with normal urine production can occur, due to reduced tubular absorption, and may carry a better prognosis than the former

Laboratory tests
Blood biochemistry
- Azotaemia can be due to pre-renal, renal, or post-renal failure
- Dehydration can lead to levels of urea and creatinine that would indicate genuine renal failure in other species; biochemistry should be performed again after adequate fluid therapy
- Failure to respond to fluid therapy suggests renal failure rather than pre-renal failure

Urinalysis
- ARF typically results in:
  - Urine creatinine: plasma creatinine low (in cat <10:1)
  - High urinary sodium (>25 mmol/l in the cat)
- SG usually elevated in pre-renal disease, but may be lowered in:
  - Concurrent renal disease
  - Fluid or diuretic administration
  - Septicaemia
  - Hepatic disease
  - Hyperkalaemia, hyperphosphataemia, acidosis
- Presence of .
  - Casts
  - Excessive protein
  - Glucose (may be stress induced, however)
  - Blood and white blood cells
  - Bacteria: should be cultured if present

Renal biopsy
- Histopathology and electron microscopy to determine viability of renal tubular basement membrane and thus prognosis

Treatment
- Prevent further renal tubular damage
  - GI absorbants, specific antidotes, diuresis
- Avoid nephrotoxic drugs, e.g. sulphonamides and aminoglycosides
  - Fluids and parenteral vitamin B_6 may be protective against nephrotoxicity when using such drugs
- Fluid therapy to dilute uraemic toxins and maintain renal perfusion and urine output
  - Correct fluid and electrolyte deficits/imbalances, avoiding overhydration
- Uraemia may damage oral and GI mucosa
  - H_2 blockers, GI prokinetics, sucralfate, force feeding if anorexic
- Anabolic steroids
  - As an appetite stimulant
  - May help to retain electrolytes and reduce protein catabolism
- Antimicrobials
  - To treat pyelonephritis
  - To prevent bacterial infection in immune compromised patients

Fluid therapy
- Careful monitoring of respiratory rate, nature and auscultation is necessary
  - Fluid therapy rates must be adjusted in light of urine output
- Diuretics may be used once rehydration is complete
  - Rabbits are less sensitive to loop diuretics than other species
- Lack of urine output within 24 hours of treatment initiation carries a grave prognosis
- Serum potassium must be monitored and hyperkalaemia controlled
- Dextrose-containing fluids may be advised in severe hyperkalaemia, to shift potassium into cells
- Peritoneal dialysis
  - May be performed (risk of damage to gut +/− peritonitis)
  - 40 ml/kg, leave for 30–40 minutes, then drain

Prevention
- Identify rabbits at risk
- Fluid therapy, e.g. perioperatively

ORGAN SYSTEMS

- Avoid nephrotoxic drug use
  - If vital, use with care
  - Concurrent fluid and diuretic therapy
  - Dose accurately: weigh patient, use small syringes, dilute drug
- Treat affected or suspected cases early and aggressively in the disease process
- Avoid obesity
- Avoid excess calcium and vitamin D in diet
- Ensure water ad libitum at all times
- Minimize stress
- Minimize exposure to excessive heat

CHRONIC RENAL FAILURE

Predisposing factors/causes
- Age related renal fibrosis
- Chronic pyelonephritis
- *Encephalitozoon cuniculi*
- High calcium diet
- High vitamin D content of diet
- Nephrolithiasis
- Nephrotoxins
- Obesity
- Amyloid deposition as a consequence of chronic inflammatory disease (abscess, endometritis, pododermatitis, etc.)

Diagnosis
History
- Age
  - Generally older rabbits

Clinical signs
- Depression
- Lethargy
- Anorexia
- GI stasis
- Weight loss
- PU/PD
- Perineal urine scalding, possibly leading to secondary myiasis
- Uraemic breath

Physical examination
- Dehydration
- Weight loss
- Changes in renal size and shape
- Oral ulceration, corneal ulceration
- Oedema, especially following fluid therapy

Laboratory findings
- Anaemia
  - Non-regenerative anaemia
  - Decreased platelet count
- Azotaemia
  - Dehydration can lead to levels of urea and creatinine that would indicate genuine renal failure in other species
  - Biochemistry should be performed again after adequate fluid therapy
- Hyperphosphataemia
- Hypercalcaemia or hypocalcaemia
- Hypokalaemia
- Isosthenuria
- Clear urine due to impaired calcium excretion and metabolic changes
- Glycosuria if significant tubular damage

Radiography
- Small or misshapen kidneys
- Soft tissue mineralization, especially devitalized tissue and aorta
- Renal mineralization or nephrolithiasis

Differential diagnosis
- Dental disease
  - Commonly causes weight loss, along with PU/PD as a result of oral ulceration
- Diabetes mellitus (rare)
- Internal abscessation
- Uterine infection
  - Metritis
  - Pyometra

Management of chronic renal failure

Dietary

Provision of a normal diet (see Clinical nutrition and gastrointestinal disorders, p. 105).

- Healthy caecal flora will utilize urea as part of the digestive process and possibly ameliorate some of the signs of uraemia
- Optimum nutrition as above, with probiotics and GI prokinetics as necessary, may assist this process
- In short term, force or assisted feeding may be necessary
- Highly palatable food sources may be helpful short term
- Fluid and electrolyte therapy
  - Parenterally or orally, as appropriate

High water content fresh food.
- Increased palatability
- Enhanced water intake

Moderate calcium intake.
- Stop any supplementation
- Minimal alfalfa intake
- See p. 117 for list of foodstuffs by calcium content

Restrict phosphate intake.
- Avoid carrots, tomatoes and banana

Other

Antimicrobials
- To treat pyelonephritis
- To prevent bacterial infection in immune compromised patients

Avoid glucocorticoids

Phosphate binders
- These may be helpful in treatment

ACE inhibitors
- Their use has not been evaluated in rabbits, but they may be a useful treatment adjunct

Anabolic steroids
- Act as an appetite stimulant

- Reduce uraemia
- May help retention of electrolytes
- Help reduce muscle catabolism

Vitamin supplementation
- B vitamins may act as an appetite stimulant, and are unlikely to do any harm in moderation, but should be present in vast excess anyway if caecotrophy is being performed
- Many supplementary foods will already contain these, so extra supplementation may not be of any benefit

Potassium supplementation
- May be advisable in cases where hypokalaemia is demonstrated

Erythropoeitin
- Useful in cases of anaemia due to CRF

LOWER URINARY TRACT DISORDERS

Special considerations in calcium metabolism
- Rabbits are different from other mammals with respect to their calcium metabolism
  - They absorb a much higher proportion of dietary calcium than other species
  - Rate of calcium excretion is also related to their dietary levels of calcium
  - Urinary fractional excretion rate for calcium is in the order of 45–60% as opposed to typical rates of 2% for other mammals
- Very large quantities of calcium (usually as calcium carbonate) can be found in rabbit urine, and the level of calcium found in the urine (assuming other factors, e.g. water consumption, are unchanged) is related to the level of calcium found in the diet

- Any condition causing urine retention in rabbits can lead to sediment accumulation in the bladder
  - This 'sludge' may be clinically silent, may irritate the urinary tract mucosa, precipitating urinary tract infections, or may form the basis for calculi, which can occur in renal pelvis, ureter, bladder or urethra
  - Clinically silent 'sand' or 'sludge' may mask true calculi
  - 'Sludge' that settles out and solidifies rather than remaining in suspension in urine, is more of a clinical problem
- Uroliths, usually of calcium carbonate, sometimes of calcium oxalate, may commonly occur
- Ammonium magnesium phosphate crystals can also occur in normal rabbit urine, and in association with abnormalities

Diagnosis
History
- Age
- Sex
- Entire or neutered?
- Any other behavioural changes, e.g. spraying
- Previous history of urinary tract problems
- Diet
- Supplements given
- Water intake and method of water provision
- Locomotor problems
- Obesity
- Environment:
  - Indoor or outdoor?
  - Litter trained or not?
  - Single or group rabbit?

Clinical signs
- Frequent small amounts of urine passed
- No urine passed
- Difficulty urinating

- Increased licking around perineal area
- Any suggestion of abdominal pain?
  - Inappetance
  - Hunched posture
- Haematuria

Physical examination
- Abdominal palpation
- Bladder, kidneys, uterus in particular
  - The bladder may be felt as an enlarged structure
  - The bladder may have a granular feel on palpation
  - Evidence of pain on bladder palpation
  - Some rabbits may strain when bladder palpated, if uroliths present
- Examination of perineal skin and external genitalia
- Assessment of body condition and localized fat deposits near vulva/penis
- Observation of rabbit walking/hopping/ jumping over objects to assess mobility
- Observation of rabbit urinating if possible

Urinalysis
- See Urinalysis, p. 83

Blood analysis
- See Azotaemia p. 75 and Electrolyte abnormalities, p. 76, to differentiate renal disease
- Unless urinary tract obstruction or bladder rupture has taken place, few if any changes may be expected
- Serology for *Encephalitozoon cuniculi*

Imaging
- Plain abdominal radiography
  - Including kidneys and entire pelvis
- Abdominal ultrasonography
  - Including bladder, uterus, kidneys
- Contrast abdominal radiography
  - IVU
  - Negative contrast bladder radiography
  - Double contrast bladder radiography

- Urethral catheterization is possible in both male and female rabbits, but may require sedation or anaesthesia
  - A 9F catheter is suitable for average sized rabbits of either sex
- Rolling the animal from side to side to move calculi around within the bladder during ultrasonography, may help to reveal them
  - Uroliths may cast a shadow or cause a reflection on ultrasonography
- Males are restrained in dorsal recumbency and the catheter advanced 1.5–4 cm into the urethra to obtain a sample
- The urethral orifice of the female is best accessed by passing the catheter along the ventral floor of the vagina with the doe in ventral recumbency

Managing obstruction, 'sludgy' urine and urolithiasis in rabbits

Note that 'sludge' and urolithiasis are different conditions, although, as many of the factors that contribute to them are the same, they may both be present at the same time.

Obstruction of lower urinary tract, i.e. urethra
Causes
- 'Sludge'
- Urethral muscle spasm
- Inflammation, fibrosis, adhesions, abscesses
- Calculi

Findings
- In all but the earliest cases of total lower urinary tract obstruction, the bladder is usually markedly palpably enlarged
- A ruptured bladder is a possible consequence of urinary tract obstruction either directly or following attempts at bladder expression or palpation, and cannot be ruled out in any case where the bladder cannot be palpated

- Such cases are usually, but not entirely exclusively, restricted to male rabbits
- Discrete calculi, or accretions of 'sludge' may cause obstruction
- Urethral muscle spasm can occur following catheterization
- Inflammation and fibrosis can occur, usually in the distal urethra, following trauma

Treatment
- Urethral muscle spasm usually responds to benzodiazepines
- Inflammation usually responds to anti-inflammatories and specific treatment, e.g. antibiotics
- If there is occlusion of the urethra then catheterization or repeated cystocentesis may be necessary pending resolution
- Fibrosis may require surgical rectification
- Urethral calculi may be retropulsed into the bladder and removed via cystotomy, 'milked' out, under GA, or retrieved via urethrotomy as necessary
  - Lithotripsy has been used in research settings, but rarely if ever in practice situations

Obstruction of upper urinary tract, i.e. ureter
Causes
- Ureteral ligation
- Ureteral calculi
- Involvement in abscess, neoplasia, adhesion, etc.

Ureteral ligation is a possible consequence of ovariohysterectomy.
- Diagnosis is based on suspicious clinical signs (abdominal pain, attempts to strain to pass urine, inappetance, shortly after ovariohysterectomy)
- This can be confirmed by exploratory laparotomy or IVU

ORGAN SYSTEMS

Ureteral calculi can occlude the ureters.
- Diagnosis is based on suspicious clinical signs, and confirmed by plain radiographs of the abdomen, IVU or exploratory surgery
- Plain radiographs may be difficult to interpret, with small uroliths often difficult to visualize especially in DV views, against radiodense material such as ingesta or vertebrae

In either case hydronephrosis and hydro-ureter may be observed on radiography, and confirmed on ultrasonography.
- Exploratory surgery will be necessary to correct the problem, either by correction of the ureteral problem, or unilateral nephrectomy in advanced cases

Note that bilateral involvement is common, and that the contralateral kidney and ureter should be closely examined and renal function of the rabbit should be investigated before nephrectomy is carried out.
- Plain radiography, ultrasonography, and an intravenous excretory pyelogram are advised, along with biochemical evaluation of renal function

Initial therapy
- The bladder should be decompressed if full, either by cystocentesis or catheterization
- The former may be easier, especially if very full, but carries the risk of potential bladder rupture
- The latter usually requires sedation, but is more effective in removing large volumes of urine from the bladder, and the ease of catheter passage can provide information about the site of obstruction
- Retropulsion of uroliths may be possible using this method
- The bladder should be lavaged repeatedly with warm saline until no suspended material can be seen, and the bladder feels empty of particulate material
- If unobstructed, or after obstruction is relieved, further investigation and treatment can take place, as above
- Diuresis with 100 ml/kg/day parenteral fluids should be administered, once urine flow has been established
- Urethral muscle spasm following catheterization can be avoided by gentle technique and the use of benzodiazepines in the anaesthetic/sedation routine

Decision making in 'sludgey' rabbits
- Excessive levels of sediment in the urine lead to 'sand' or 'sludge' forming on the cranioventral floor of the bladder
  - Diets high in calcium and protein, and low fluid intakes increase the density of the sediment in the urine
  - Physical inactivity in cage bound animals may predispose to settlement of the sediment
- Radiodense material in the bladder may be seen on radiographs of normal, clinically healthy rabbits
- Crystals do not necessarily mean calculi have formed
  - No treatment is required if the rabbit is otherwise without symptoms
  - If other symptoms are present, treatment will be necessary
- Any calcium supplementation should be withdrawn, or the dose modified
  - Alfalfa and calcium-rich foodstuffs should be withdrawn, or fed in moderation
  - Protein-rich foodstuffs should be avoided

Encourage water intake
- Fresh grass as opposed to hay or dried grass
  - Fresh grass first thing in the morning is wet with dew; allow rabbit outside earlier
- Ad libitum fresh green leafy vegetation

- Soak or steam hay, or wet the grass and other foods
  ○ (Do not allow the hay to become mouldy)
- Flavoured water (fruit juice, etc.)
  ○ May encourage water intake
  ○ May also discourage drinking by some rabbits
  ○ May lead to bacterial growth in the water
- Some plants may have mild diuretic properties, e.g. Yarrow, plantain, dandelion, goosegrass
- Subcutaneous fluids
  ○ Regular administration of SC fluids has helped in some cases
  ○ These may be given by the owner long term

Diuretics
- Bendrofluazide 600 µg/kg PO once a day in the mornings has been suggested to reduce calcium oxalate urolithiasis and calcium-rich 'sludge' formation
  ○ Bendrofluazide is used as a calcium-retaining diuretic in human patients with osteoporotic disease
- Although soft tissue mineralization has not been reported with this regime, this is a potential risk, and the levels of calcium in the diet (and thus the urine) should be addressed

Bethanechol
- May improve bladder tone and increase sediment voidance

Encourage mobility
- Obese rabbits may be more at risk
- Inactive rabbits may be more at risk
- Rabbits that are unable to assume a normal urinating posture are more at risk
- Regular ballottement of the abdomen may help to minimize settling of the sediment
- Emptying of the bladder under sedation or GA, with the rabbit held vertically

upright, may help in fully emptying the bladder of 'sludge' and small uroliths
  ○ Any condition that reduces the ability to posture to or express urine, risks incomplete bladder emptying and 'sludge' accumulation
  ○ Any mobility disorder, stiffness, obesity, etc., should be investigated and treatment attempted
- In recalcitrant cases, bladder lavage by catheterization and repeated flushing with warm saline, or via cystotomy, may be required
- Note that the presence of suture material within the bladder can act as a nidus for future calculus formation, and should be avoided, by using rapidly absorbed, fine suture material, such as Poliglecaprone 25 (Monocryl, Ethicon) or Polyglactin 912 (Vicryl, Ethicon)
- Recurrence of the problem, even after surgery, is likely, if preventative measures are not taken.

Other agents
- Calcium oxalate crystalluria and calculi may be related to intake of oxalates from plants (See Nutritional requirements of rabbits, p. 105)
- Lack of oxalobacter in the gut may occur, and predispose to oxalate urolithiasis by reduced oxalate breakdown
  ○ In humans with genetic or acquired hyperoxaluria and renal mineralization or uroliths *Oxalobacter formigenes* probiotic formulations are being used to colonise the GIT with oxalate reducing bacteria
- *NB*: Dietary acidification is of no benefit, and is difficult or impossible to achieve without feeding a highly inappropriate diet
- Potassium citrate orally has been suggested for rabbits with calcium oxalate urolithiasis to reduce urinary calcium concentration

ORGAN SYSTEMS

Lower urinary tract infection

- Primary urinary tract infection is moderately uncommon
  - Diagnosis and treatment have been covered under infection as a cause of renal disease
  - The most effective test is bacterial culture and sensitivity, and/or cytology for white cells, bacteria and casts, from cystocentesed urine
- Antibiotic administration should be based on bacterial culture and sensitivity, and continued for 7 days after the resolution of clinical signs (for a minimum of 4 weeks in cases of confirmed bacterial cystitis, and 10 days where no bacteria are detected)
- 'Sludge' in the urinary tract can cause urethral irritation and predispose to infection
- Urinary tract infection secondary to calculi is more common, and should be treated as above, together with measures to control the crystalluria/uroliths
- There may be some benefit to the use of N-acetyl-D-glucosamine products or cranberry extract products to decrease bacterial attachment to the bladder mucosa
- Dandelions, as well as having a high water content, are believed to have a mild diuretic effect
- As for urolithiasis, free and dietary water intake should be increased

Urinary incontinence

- *Encephalitozoon cuniculi*
  - See p. 101
- Toxoplasmosis
  - Can cause paresis, but is much less common
- Other CNS lesions may cause hindlimb paresis:
  - Neoplasia
  - Abscesses
  - Listeriosis
  - Spinal trauma due to

- – Road traffic collision, predation, sudden kicking out of back legs
- – Lumbar vertebral subluxation at L6/L7
- Need to differentiate LMN and UMN bladder for treatment regime and prognosis
- May require full neurological examination, radiography and myelography to fully evaluate
- Atonic bladders may benefit from treatment with bethanecol
- Urethritis, cystitis and urinary tract 'sludge' may mimic incontinence

Urethral incompetence in speyed female rabbits

- Similar clinical picture to that in the speyed bitch
- Urinary incontinence has occasionally been described following ovariohysterectomy
- Appears to respond to phenylpropanolamine (Propalin, Vetoquinol) or Estriol (Incurin, Intervet)

URINE SCALDING OF PERINEAL SKIN

- Perineal inflammation due to urine scald is a multifactorial disease syndrome
  - In turn, it can create further problems

Factors in its development
Urinary tract, etc., disorders
- Urinary incontinence
- Overflowing bladder (severe PU/PD, LMN bladder)
- Cystitis
- Urine 'sludge'
- Urolithiasis
- *Encephalitozoon cuniculi*

Problems affecting ability to urinate away from body
- Obesity or large skin folds

- External genitalia inflammation, pain or deformity
  - Wounds
  - *Treponema cuniculi*
- *Encephalitozoon cuniculi*
- Inability to stand properly
  - e.g. Spinal lesion
  - Hindlimb arthritis
  - Ulcerative pododermatitis
  - Cage too small to position properly

Problems affecting ability to keep area clean

- Dental disease
- Painful skin
- Inability to raise hind end from ground easily
- Unhygienic/damp bedding

Other problems causing perineal lesions

- Flystrike
- Caecotroph accumulation

- Vaginal discharge
- Fur accumulation (long furred breeds, grooming problems)

Sequelae of perineal urine scald

- Flystrike
- Reluctance to ingest caecotrophs leading to accumulation
- Worsening of condition as skin is not kept clean
- Reluctance to move due to pain
  - Resulting in exacerbation of obesity, pododermatitis, etc.
- Immune suppression, anaemia, secondary diseases

Treatment

- Treat local skin inflammation symptomatically
  - Investigate and treat underlying factors
  - May require skin fold resection if there is obesity or loose skin

DISORDERS OF THE GENITAL SYSTEM

DISORDERS OF THE MALE GENITAL TRACT

Many pet male rabbits are castrated, but single pet males are common and even some in pairs or groups may be entire. Infertility is covered elsewhere (pp. 42, 45).

Testes

Congenital abnormalities

- Intersex (presence of one testis and one ovary, both intra-abdominal) has been reported

Trauma

- Very common in group-housed entire bucks
- Especially common in presence of doe
- Injuries often specifically directed at testes, as bucks kick out at underside of attacker

Neoplasia

- Seminomas, Sertoli cell tumours, teratomas, interstial cell carcinomas have been reported
- Epididymal cysts can occur, and be difficult to differentiate from the above on palpation
- Incidence of neoplasia is increased in cryptorchid rabbits
- Castration is the usual treatment of choice
- Differentiation from abscesses is possible by biopsy, but as castration is appropriate for either condition, excisional biopsies are preferred
- Bilateral neoplasia has been reported; for this, if for no other reason, bilateral castration and histopathology is advised

Abscesses/orchitis/epidydmitis

- Following local trauma, e.g. fighting most commonly

ORGAN SYSTEMS

- Haematogenous spread from other foci of infection is less common
- Castration is curative
- Medical management is unlikely to result in functional testis
- *Pasteurella multocida* and *Treponema cuniculi* may be isolated

Cryptorchidism

- Misdiagnosis of cryptorchidism is common, as rabbits commonly retract their testes through their large, open inguinal canal when stressed, or during illness or malnutrition
  - Allowing the rabbit to relax, trancing/hypnosis, or sedation/anaesthesia, followed by placing the rabbit vertically upright and massaging the lower abdomen, may be necessary to encourage the testes to descend
- True cryptorchid rabbits are very rare
  - In genuine cryptorchid rabbits, the scrotal sac remains undeveloped on the affected side(s)
  - Traumatic castration, or traumatic scrotal resection, or necrosis during fighting, and subsequent scarring of the site may mimic this appearance
- Cryptorchid rabbits appear more susceptible to testicular neoplasia, and histopathology of the testes should be performed
- There may be a hereditary component; such rabbits and their siblings, parents and offspring should not be bred from

Myxomatosis

- In the early stages of myxomatosis, oedema of the scrotal skin may be the only clinical sign
  - In later stages, the pathological changes to the face are nearly always pathognomonic, but examination for oedema and inflammation of scrotal and preputial skin may help confirm the diagnosis

Penis/prepuce
Trauma and inflammation

- Trauma and subsequent deformation of the penis and prepuce can be as a result of:
  - Fighting
  - Following paramphimosis
  - Self-trauma following urolithiasis
  - Mutilation by parents when young kit
- Early intervention and good surgical alignment, with minimization of fibrosis are ideal
- Poor penile conformation can predispose to further trauma or self trauma, drying of the tip of the penis, and urine scalding
- Paramphimosis has commonly been reported following castration (also see below)
  - This may be due to interference with the penile suspensory ligament
  - Most such cases resolve with time, and symptomatic treatment to avoid drying of the penis is all that is required until that time
  - In severe cases, partial amputation may be necessary

Fur entanglement

- Fur entrapment of the penis is much less common than in the chinchilla (*Chinchilla lanigera*), but does occasionally occur, especially in long-haired rabbits
- Removal of the fur, and symptomatic treatment are necessary

Urethral urolithiasis

- Uroliths can form very distally in the urethra and lead to self trauma
  - Rabbits can also overgroom and self traumatize due to urinary tract obstruction anywhere along the urethra

- Treatment of the underlying cause and the resultant inflammation require appropriate symptomatic therapy

Paramphimosis and sequelae
- A syndrome of paramphimosis following castration has been widely reported
- There does not appear to be any correlation with anaesthetic agents used, as is the case in the horse, nor with the method of castration
- Minor trauma, leading to interference with nerve or vascular supply to the musculature of the area, is thought to be the cause
- Most cases resolve within a matter of hours, occasionally days, and should be kept moist until they do so
- Avoidance of irritant substrates, e.g. sawdust, is advised

Accessory sex glands
- Male rabbits possess prostate glands, coagulating glands, bulbourethral glands and vesicular glands associated with the urogenital system
  - Anal glands are also found, just inside the anus.
- Clinically silent squamous metaplasia and hyperplastic changes of the prostate and vesicular glands were reported in significant numbers of NZW and Dutch rabbits sampled at post mortem
  - It is extremely rare for there to be any clinical problems involving these accessory glands
- Preputial and inguinal glands are found in the dermis around the prepuce, and either side of the penis, respectively
  - The inguinal glands in particular can become impacted with exudates, and may contribute to flystrike
  - Simple cleaning is usually sufficient, with symptomatic treatment as necessary for inflammation or infection

External genital skin
Urine scald
- Usually secondary to urine outflow disorder, mobility disorder, or penile malpositioning
- (See Urinary tract disease, p. 150)

Treponema paraluis-cuniculi ('rabbit syphilis' or 'vent disease')
Epidemiology
- Not zoonotic
- Transmitted venereally between rabbits and vertically at parturition and lactation
- Pain may inhibit mating, reducing fertility
- May remain asymptomatic until animal is stressed
- Once infected, clinical signs are self-limiting, but animal is a carrier
- Recovered bucks have star shaped scars on scrotum
- Long incubation periods (10–16 weeks)

Clinical findings
- Lesions start as reddened areas on the genitals that progresses to oedema, vesicles, ulceration and scabbing around perineum/genitalia
- Grooming activity spreads disease to face
- Vesicles burst and develop into crusting lesions
- Inguinal lymph nodes may become enlarged

Diagnosis
- Histopathology
- Silver stains on affected tissues
- Dark field microscopy on scrapings of tissues
- Human Treponema serology testing kits (25% of healthy rabbits are seropositive)

Differential diagnosis
- Dermatophytosis
- Myxomatosis

ORGAN SYSTEMS

ORGAN SYSTEMS

- Trauma of face through pushing nose through cage bars or wire
- Recto-anal papillomas

Treatment
- Appropriate antibiotics
  - Historically penicillins
  - Safer drugs now available
  - See Treponemiasis, p. 193

Myxomatosis
- See p. 188
- Other clinical signs usually pathognomonic

DISORDERS OF THE FEMALE GENITAL TRACT AND MAMMARY GLANDS

Ovarohysterectomy of all female rabbits not intended for breeding is strongly advised, given the high incidence of uterine adenocarcinoma in entire female rabbits. However, a relatively low proportion of female rabbits are speyed, in contrast to the feline situation.

Ovaries
- Intersex (presence of one testis and one ovary) has been reported
- Neoplasia
  - Primary, e.g. ovarian haemangioma
  - Local spread/involvement from uterus
- Abscesses
  - *Pasteurella multocida* abscesses
- Cysts
  - Rare

Clinical signs
- Abdominal enlargement
- Alopecia may be seen

Diagnosis
- Biopsy +/– aspiration of cystic fluid
  - (At exploratory laparotomy or ultrasound guided)

- As ovariectomy/ovarohysterectomy is the treatment of choice, excisional biopsies are preferred
  - Samples can be submitted for histopathology, and culture and sensitivity
  - Survey radiography is advised to check for metastases/other foci of infection

Uterus
Dystocia
- Kindling problems rare in rabbits
- Most common in obese does not bred until late in life
- Management as for other species

Uterine prolapse
- Rare complication of dystocia
- Treatment by lubrication, reduction and ovariohysterectomy

Extra-uterine pregnancy
- Relatively common
- Often subclinical
- Often trauma related
- Release of fertilized ovum of fetus into abdominal cavity, or ruptured uterus

Pregnancy toxaemia
- Uncommon
- Usually seen in last week of pregnancy
  - Often in primaparous does
- Usually in obese does
  - Can occur in pseudopregnancy and post-partum does
- Combination of high energy requirements and decreased GIT space
  - Acute mobilization of fat reserves leading to hepatic lipidosis
  - Lethargy, anorexia, hypersalivation
  - Ketones in blood, urine and acetone smell on breath
  - Urine pH becomes acidic (6 or even lower)
- May develop dyspnoea, seizures, coma, death
- May abort spontaneously, in which case better prognosis

Supportive treatment
- Fluids containing glucose/complex polysaccharides
- Nutritional support
- Short acting glucocorticoids
- Calcium supplementation (parenteral or oral)
- Ovariohysterectomy when stable
- Induce abortion

Prevention
- Avoid obesity in breeding does
- Increase exercise in breeding does
- Avoid stress or other factors leading to anorexia

Endometritis
- *Pasteurella multocida, Staphylococcus aureus* and other bacteria
  - Haematogenous spread or infection during mating
  - Post-partum metritis also seen
  - May be associated with hypervitaminosis A
- Stillbirth and metritis seen following uterine torsion
- Reduced fertility in breeding does
- May develop into pyometra
  - Can also occur in unmated does, especially pseudopregnant ones

Clinical signs
- Weakness, anorexia, creamy vaginal discharge, PU/PD

Diagnosis
- May develop into abscessation of uterus or ovaries
- May be palpably enlarged uterus (care with abdominal palpation, as uterus may rupture)
- May lead to marked leucocytosis (heterophilia)
- Bacteria present in vaginal discharge

Treatment
- Some cases may respond to medical treatment

- Otherwise stabilize rabbit and ovariohysterectomy

Endometrial hyperplasia
- Natural ageing process
  - Uterine endometrial glandular tissue becomes hyperplastic with age
  - Progression to polyp formation or metritis
  - May result in uterine adenocarcinoma
  - May be induced by inactive cystic ovaries
- Clinical signs may include:
  - Reduced fertility
  - Abdominal pain
  - Anorexia
  - Flystrike
  - Haematuria at end of micturition, often clotted, sometimes intermittent
  - Cystic mammary changes

Diagnosis
- Abdominal radiography
- Abdominal ultrasonography

Treatment
- Ovariohysterectomy

Uterine neoplasia
- Uterine adenocarcinoma most common
- Can occur from 2 years of age
- May be clinically silent until far advanced
- May be behavioural changes, especially aggression
- May be a progression of endometrial hyperplasia
- May alternatively be due to ageing changes/decreased oestrogens
  - (Decreased cellularity, increased collagen deposition in uterus)
- Most common neoplasm of pet rabbits
- May be increased incidence in Tan, French silver, Havana and Dutch rabbits
- Incidence independent of breeding history
- Insidious development
- Can metastasize to lungs, liver, brain, bone, spleen and mammary gland

ORGAN SYSTEMS

- Local spread within abdomen can occur
- May see dyspnoea or ascites if metastasis/spread
- Clinical signs and diagnosis as for endometrial hyperplasia, p. 169

Treatment
- Ovarohysterectomy (ensure entire uterus removed)
- Examine for local spread in abdomen
- Survey (thoracic) radiography to examine for metastasis
- Re-examine for metastasis every 3–6 months for 1–2 years

Prognosis
- Good if no local or distant spread
  ○ Metastasis unlikely if no local spread and no serosal ulceration
  ○ Other neoplasia is less common, e.g. leiomyoma, and should be treated similarly, with definite diagnosis and prognosis determined on histopathology

Endometrial venous aneurysm
- Similar presentation to that of uterine adenocarcinoma
- Aetiology unknown
- Histology required to differentiate
- May develop large, blood-filled uterus
- May lead to life threatening blood loss

Treatment
- Ovariohysterectomy

Hydrometra/mucometra
- Uterus full of fluid
- Due to influence of progesterone in pseudopregnancy
  ○ Stimulates uterine fluid secretion
  ○ Stimulates cervical closure
- If corpus luteum remains, uterus fills with fluid

Clinical signs
- Abdominal enlargement

- Fluid filled abdomen similar to ascites
- Fluid has low relative density (SG), moderate protein and low cellularity

Diagnosis
- Abdominal radiography
- Abdominal ultrasound
- Exploratory laparotomy

Treatment
- Ovariohysterectomy
- Medical management not advised, as even if effective, recurrence is very likely

Uterine torsion
- Rare
- Always in association with uterine enlargement due to pregnancy, pyometra, hydrometra or adenocarcinoma
- Rabbit often presents in extreme shock
- Treat underlying cause
- Stabilize rabbit for surgery

Treatment
- Ovariohysterectomy

Vagina/vulva
- *Pasteurella multocida* can be found in the vagina, and may cause vulvo-vaginitis

Vaginal prolapse
- Can occur at times of sexual receptivity
  ○ Genetic predisposition suspected
- Accompanied by severe haemorrhage and shock
  ○ Supportive care followed by replacement or resection of affected tissues
- Differential diagnosis
  ○ Vaginal polyps can also occur

Mammary glands
Bacterial mastitis
- Bacterial infection in lactating does (commonly *Staphylococcus aureus*, *Streptococcus* spp. and *Pasteurella* spp.)
- Haematogenous spread
- Local infection via dirty bedding

- Glands are hot and painful
- Milk retention in pseudopregnancy may also lead to mastitis
- Severe cases may lead to sepsis and debility

Treatment
- Antibiosis
- Supportive care (fluids, nutrition)
- Analgesia
- Removal of kits to prevent starvation or bacterial enteritis
- Prolactin inhibitors (Galastop) to reduce lactation
- Warm compresses applied to mammary glands
- Drainage of abscesses
- Surgical excision necessary in severe cases

Cystic mastitis
- Older does (usually 3 years plus)
- Usually non-breeding entire does
- Does may show behavioural signs of pseudopregnancy
- Often occurs concurrently with endometrial hyperplasia or uterine adenocarcinoma
- Large, bluish cysts in one or more glands
- May be serous, sometimes brown tinged discharge from nipple
- Gland is not hot or painful

Treatment
- Local treatment unnecessary
- Usually regresses following ovariohysterectomy
- Surgical excision if no resolution in 3–4 weeks
- If untreated, can progress to benign and malignant neoplasia

Mammary neoplasia
- Benign mixed adenoma
- Mammary papilloma
- Mammary adenocarcinoma
- Most common in entire does over 3 years of age

- May metastasize, to regional lymph nodes or distant organs, e.g. lungs; thoracic radiography advised as for uterine adenocarcinoma

Management
- As in the dog or cat
- Ovariohysterectomy recommended in conjunction with surgical removal, as such patients also often have uterine adenocarcinomas

Mammary dysplasia
- Secondary to prolactin secreting pituitary adenomas
- Reported in aged, primaparous NZW rabbits

External genital skin
Rabbit syphilis
- *Treponema paraluis-cuniculi*
- Transmitted venereally between rabbits
- Pain may inhibit mating, reducing fertility
- May remain asymptomatic until animal is stressed
- Once infected, clinical signs are self-limiting, but animal is a carrier
- Lesions start as reddened areas that progress to oedema, vesicles, ulceration and scabbing around perineum and genitalia
- Grooming activity spreads disease to face
  o Inguinal lymph nodes may become enlarged
- Infected does have increased incidence of metritis, placental retention and neonatal deaths

Diagnosis
- Clinical signs
- Histopathology
- Silver stains on affected tissues
- Dark field microscopy on scrapings of tissues
- Human *Treponema* serology testing kits (25% of healthy rabbits are seropositive)

ORGAN SYSTEMS

Differential diagnosis
- Dermatophytosis
- Myxomatosis

Treatment
- Appropriate antibiotics
  - Penicillins traditionally used
  - Safer alternatives available
  - See also Treponemiasis, p. 193

PSEUDOPREGNANCY

Physiological endocrine disturbance rather than an endocrinopathy. Very common in pet rabbits.

Aetiology/risk factors
- Due to increased prolactin levels, arising from ovulation without conception
  - As rabbits are induced ovulators, this can occur following unsuccessful mating, an infertile male, excitement caused by the proximity of entire bucks, mounting by another doe or 'pair bonding' with an owner or toy
- Any entire female rabbit may develop this condition
  - Those kept with another female, or strongly bonded to an owner, as well as those exposed to males (entire, vasectomized or recently castrated) are most at risk

Diagnosis
- Clinical signs include:
  - Mammary gland hyperplasia
  - Milk secretion
  - Fur removal from mammary regions, hips and dewlap
  - Nest making
  - Aggression and increased territoriality towards rabbits, humans and other animals
- Duration is 15–18 days

History and physical examination
- There may be a history of recent ovulatory behaviour as noted above, but this may not have been observed
- Any entire female of reproductive age may develop this condition

Management
- Self limiting
- Prevention of recurrence by ovariohysterectomy
- Proligestone (Delvosteron, Intervet) at 30 mg/kg SC injection
- Cabergoline (Galastop, Boehringer Ingelheim) 5 μg/kg once daily for 4–6 days, especially to relieve lactational signs
  - Repeated treatment (i.e. every time the rabbit is in oestrus) would be necessary, and this option, if used, is best followed by ovariohysterectomy

Complications
- Persistent mammary hyperplasia and lactation may lead to mastitis
- Persistent or recurrent pseudopregnancy can lead to hydrometra, as progesterone stimulates cervical closure and uterine fluid secretion
- Excessive fur pulling may contribute to the development of anorexia and reduced GI motility

DISEASES OF THE BLOOD, HAEMATOPOIETIC AND IMMUNE SYSTEMS

BLOOD CLOTTING DISORDERS

Clotting mechanisms and coagulation disorders have been well studied in rabbits both as a model for human coagulation disorders and for investigations into the effects of anticoagulant rodenticides.

Although an inherited bleeding disorder similar to von Willebrand's disease has been identified in an inbred strain of laboratory rabbits, other inherited or acquired bleeding disorders appear to be rare.

- Rodenticide poisoning
  - Rabbits have a variable and genetically determined resistance to warfarin toxicity
- VHD
- DIC as a consequence of septicaemia or toxaemia

LYMPHOMA

Lymphoproliferative disease is reasonably common in rabbits, and the occurrence of the disease in groups of related rabbits has led to suggestions regarding a genetic or viral aetiology. In one laboratory strain of 'wire-hair' rabbits a single autosomal recessive gene is responsible.

- Various forms of lymphoma have been described (multicentric, cutaneous, leukaemic, thymoma), and there have been many papers using the rabbit as an experimental model for chemotherapeutic protocols for lymphoma in humans
- In the veterinary clinical literature much of the published work refers to individual cases or anecdotal reports
  - There are reports of long term remissions following excision of thymic lymphosarcomas
  - Chemotherapeutics may have a place, but there is a significant risk in the non-specific pathogen-free pet rabbit population of immunosuppressive therapies causing reactivation of dormant infections such as encephalitozoonosis or pasteurellosis
- The reader is referred to Huston and Quesenberry (2004) for further information

ORGAN SYSTEMS

SECTION 4
INFECTIOUS DISEASES

BORDETELLOSIS

EPIDEMIOLOGY

- *Bordetella bronchiseptica*
- As a single agent infection causes only mild disease
  - However, can be an important copathogen with *Pasteurella*
- Commonly isolated from many other mammalian species, e.g. man, cat, dog, guinea pig
- Common commensal inhabitant of nares and bronchi in adults
- Prevalence increases with age
- (Can cause serious lower respiratory tract infection in guinea pigs)

ROUTE

Passed via respiratory route from animal to animal including cross species.

PATHOGENESIS

- Induces ciliostasis
- Reduces clearance of mucus
- Reduces macrophage activity
- Cytotoxic strains enhance mucosal colonization by toxigenic *Pasteurella*

CLINICAL FINDINGS

- Serous nasal discharge, often self-limiting

- In kits, weanlings and immunocompromised animals (animals on immunosuppressive drug treatments or with concurrent disease) can progress to bronchopneumonia and pleuritis

DIFFERENTIAL DIAGNOSIS

- Pasteurellosis
- Inhaled irritants
- Early myxomatosis

DIAGNOSIS

- Bacteriologic culture and sensitivity from deep nasal swab or bronchoalveolar lavage

THERAPY

Antibiosis
- Fluoroquinolones
- Tetracyclines
- Potentiated sulphonamides

CONTROL

- Specific control measures not warranted
- Ensure stress and irritant-free environment

CALICIVIRUS INFECTION

(Viral haemorrhagic disease (VHD), rabbit haemorrhagic disease (RHD))
- New viral disease in 1984
- Similar but distinct calicivirus in European hares several years earlier, and also distinct apathogenic rabbit calicivirus in Italy that may predate VHD
- Spread rapidly between commercial Chinese rabbitries and across continent
  - Reached Eastern Europe in 1988

○ Reached entire European continent by 1989
○ To Mexico through exported Chinese meat
○ Reached UK in 1992; notifiable between 1991 and 1996

EPIDEMIOLOGY

• Clinical disease only in *Oryctolagus cuniculus*
• Kits below 4–6 weeks of age have an innate immunity, independent of mother's disease status
• Rabbits over 8 weeks of age fully susceptible
• Experimental inoculation leads to death 3–4 days after infection
• In colony outbreaks, mortality peaks rapidly (at 2–3 days after initial deaths) and the outbreak lasts 1–2 weeks
• Mortality within an infected colony can be 90–100%
  ○ Some wild UK colonies seem to have better resistance and only suffer 25–50% mortality
• Endemic and widespread within the UK, with sporadic outbreaks and often unreported deaths
• Wild colonies have cyclical outbreaks every 2–3 years

ROUTE

• Direct (mutual grooming)
• Insect vectors
  ○ Mosquitoes/fleas via direct transfer of viraemic blood
  ○ Blowflies retain virus for 9 days after feeding on infected carcass, and excrete virus in their faeces
• Predator vectors
  ○ Virus shed in fox/cat faeces after eating infected carcass

• Fomites
  ○ Virus extremely stable
  ○ Up to 105 days on cloth
  ○ > 1 month at 22°C

PATHOGENESIS

• Acute necrotizing hepatosplenitis
• Release of intrahepatocytic clotting factors into the circulation
• Disseminated intravascular coagulation leads to thrombus formation
  ○ Thrombi in respiratory tract or kidneys may rupture vessels and lead to overt external haemorrhage
  ○ Thrombi in CNS may lead to tremors or seizures
  ○ Thrombi in heart or major respiratory vessels may simply lead to sudden death with no outward signs
• Animals without thrombi in critical vessels may survive long enough to develop liver failure

CLINICAL FINDINGS

• Often simply found dead, commonly in opisthotonos
• Occasionally animals found quiet, lethargic, pyrexic and hyperventilating
• Blood pressure in peripheral veins is usually extremely low, making blood sampling or fluid therapy difficult
• Develops within hours to pallor, shock and collapse
• Bleeding from vulva or foamy blood at nares may be present
• Subacute cases present with hepatic failure – jaundice and ascites
• Very occasional cases survive the liver failure, and hepatic regeneration can occur

DIFFERENTIAL DIAGNOSIS

- General differentials of sudden death
  - (?Anthrax – sudden death with haemorrhage)
- General differentials of hepatic failure
  - Hepatic coccidiosis in weanlings

DIAGNOSIS

- Vaccination status
- Clinical signs and colony/wildlife history
- Liver enzyme abnormalities and altered clotting (fibrin thrombi, decreased platelets) on blood samples
- Post-mortem examination
  - Liver usually (though not always) enlarged and friable; marked lobular pattern
  - haemorrhages in multiple organs, foamy blood in bronchi and trachea
  - segmental catarrhal enteritis
  - histopathologic hepatosplenic necrosis
- Confirmatory tests available
  - PCR
  - ELISA
  - Haemagglutination
  - Electron microscopy

THERAPY

- General supportive care, but with extremely poor prognosis
- Euthanasia on welfare and epidemiological grounds is usually indicated

CONTROL

- Inactivated (killed) VHD virus vaccine is licensed
- If vaccinating rabbits less than 10 weeks old it is necessary to repeat after that age as innate immunity may overcome vaccine antigen
- Good immunity but high incidence of 'vaccine reactions'
  - Local inflammatory swellings
  - Systemically unwell 2–5 days post vaccination
  - Possibly responses to oil adjuvant
- Attenuated VHD vaccines difficult to produce as virus does not grow well in cell culture
- Live recombinant vaccines (VHD protein in attenuated myxomavirus) being researched to give dual protection from single agent

COCCIDIOSIS

EPIDEMIOLOGY

Eimeria spp.
- Extremely common
- In pet situations usually only a clinical problem in few weeks after acquisition
- Important economic factor in breeding colonies

Twelve or more Eimeria species identified (see Table 4.1)
- Most healthy rabbits have two or more species present

- Rabbits which recover from infection develop strong immunity to that species but not cross immunity to other Eimeria

Coccidiosis can be subdivided into 'hepatic' and 'intestinal' forms
- Both types can be present at once

ROUTE

- Faeco-oral (ingested on contaminated feed)

INFECTIOUS DISEASES

INFECTIOUS DISEASES

Table 4.1 Characteristics of various *Eimeria* species of coccidia affecting rabbits

Species	Relative pathogenicity (variable within species)	Characteristic size and shape of oocyst	Description of oocysts to assist differentiation	Site of multiplication/ pathologic effect	Pre-patent period (days)
Eimeria stiedai	++++	37 × 20 μm² Ellipsoid	Smooth wall; pale yellow colour; wide, thin micropyle; no residual body; sporocyst with terminal knob (stiedai body)	Mesenteric lymph node; biliary epithelia	15–19
E. intestinalis	++++	27 × 18 μm² Ellipsoid	Smooth wall; yellow colour; micropyle present; large residual body	Ileum	10
E. magna	++++	35 × 24 μm² Ovoid/ellipsoid	Brown wall; micropyle with lip/wings; large residual body	Jejunum	6–7
E. flavescens	++++	32 × 21 μm² Ellipsoid	Smooth wall; light yellow colour; prominent micropyle; no residual body	Ileum, caecum, colon	9
E. irresidua	+++	38 × 26 μm² Ovoid	Smooth wall; light yellow colour; prominent micropyle; small residual body	Small intestine	7–8
E. neoleporis	+++	39 × 20 μm² Elongate ellipsoid	Smooth wall; yellow colour; distinct micropyle; no residual body.	Small intestine, caecum	12
E. coecicola	++	29 × 18 μm² Ellipsoid/oblong	Smooth wall; yellow colour; micropyle present; no residual body	Jejunum, ileum	9–10
E. media	++	31 × 18 μm² Ellipsoid	Smooth, thick, light pink wall; micropyle present; large residual body	Small and large intestine	6–7
E. matsubayashii	+	25 × 18 μm² Ovoid	Smooth wall; light colour; no residual body	Small intestine caecum	7
E. perforans	+/−	21 × 15 μm² Ellipsoid	Smooth wall; colourless; indistinct micropyle; small residual body	Small intestine	5
E. exigua	−	15 × 13 μm² Ovoid	Smooth wall; indistinct micropyle; no residual body	?	?
E. nagpurensis	−	23 × 13 μm² Barrel shaped	Smooth, colourless wall; no micropyle; no residual body	?	?

Sources: Okerman (1994); Pakes & Gerrity (1994); Jenkins (1997, 2004a).

- Oocysts need 2 days or more (depending on species) outside host to sporulate before becoming infective
  - Therefore oocysts in caecotrophs do not contribute to reinfection
- Remain infective on soil or vegetation for several years unless dessicated
  - Could be introduced to domestic animals through contaminated fresh vegetation (grass, weeds) used as food

PATHOGENESIS

- Oocyst ingested on food material
- Oocyst wall broken down in duodenum releasing sporozoites
- Sporozoites invade epithelial cells
- Complex life cycle leading to release of oocysts from the epithelial surface

Hepatic
- *Eimeria stiedai* only
- Most adult rabbits have a strong immunity
- Young rabbits can be highly susceptible
- Sporozoites in duodenum penetrate intestinal mucosa and are transferred either via blood or in macrophages in the lymphatic system
- Replication in mesenteric lymph nodes
  - Schizont stages can be seen on impression cytology/histopathology
- Transported via portal circulation to liver
- Infect epithelial cells of bile ducts and gall bladder
- Oocysts begin to be released into bile ducts 15 days post infection
  - Shedding continues for 10–14 days
- Sheer volume of oocysts produced turns bile cloudy and sludgy, and biliary obstruction follows
- Liver becomes enlarged and fibrotic
  - Thickening of gall bladder and bile ducts
  - 'Abscesses' up to 5 mm in diameter which exude cloudy bile when cut
  - Microscopy of bile reveals oocysts

Intestinal
- Eleven or more intestinal *Eimeria* species
- Vary greatly in pathogenicity and site of pathologic effect
- Species most commonly associated with clinical disease:
  - *Eimeria perforans*
  - *Eimeria magna*
  - *Eimeria media*
  - *Eimeria irresidua*

Clinical disease is most prevalent in young growing rabbits, partly because the major clinical sign – stunting – is only important at this stage.
- Sporozoites penetrate small intestinal epithelium
- Two asexual developmental stages
- Limited to jejunum and ileum, and occasionally caecum
- Oocysts in faeces 5–12 days post infection (depending on species)
- Inflammatory response leads to hyperaemia, oedema, ulceration and haemorrhage
- Mucosal damage allows secondary bacterial (*Escherichia coli*) infection

CLINICAL FINDINGS

- Stunting
- Weight loss
- Lethargy

Hepatic
- Ascites
- Jaundice
- Anorexia
- Death

Intestinal
- Mild intermittent diarrhoea
  - May have mucus or blood
- Dehydration
- Secondary bacterial infections
- Intussusception/rectal prolapse
- Death

DIFFERENTIAL DIAGNOSIS

Hepatic
• Theoretically other causes (toxic, congenital) of liver failure/ascites
• In practice, ascites or jaundice in a weanling rabbit is virtually pathognomonic

Intestinal
• Other causes (dietary, viral, bacterial) of diarrhoea
  ○ Often difficult to determine the primary pathogen as many colibacillosis cases will have incidental coccidia present, whilst coccidiosis cases commonly have secondary *Escherichia coli* involvement
• Mucoid enteropathy

DIAGNOSIS

Live animal
Demonstration of oocysts in faeces
• Could be incidental finding
• Need to confirm likelihood of clinically significant infection
  ○ Extremely high numbers of oocysts
  ○ Moderately high numbers of a recognized pathogenic species
  ○ Confirmed presence of *E. stiedai* in conjunction with hepatic signs
• Biochemistry may help confirm the presence of liver disease
  ○ AST, LDH, ALT
  ○ Bilirubin
  ○ Bile acids

Post-mortem findings
• See descriptions under Pathogenesis above
• Microscopical examination of scrapings of ileal mucosa, impression smears of mesenteric lymph nodes or bile material reveals developmental stages or oocysts

THERAPY

Licensed (UK) products for in-feed use are not good once clinical disease is established as appetite suppression is an early clinical sign.

• Various anti-coccidial agents are available
  ○ Sulphonamides
    — Useful since they also have effects against concurrent bacterial involvement
    — Palatable human paediatric formulations (with trimethoprim) available
    — Variable resistance of *Eimeria* strains to individual sulpha drugs
    — Sulphaquinoxaline most effective, but only available in large quantity poultry formulations
  ○ Amprolium
    — Available (UK) in small volumes as product licensed for pigeons
  ○ Toltrazuril
    — More reliably effective than other options

CONTROL

Managemental
• Prevent access to faeces of over 2 days old
  ○ Wash grass/vegetables before feeding
  ○ Avoid access of susceptible rabbits to contaminated grazing
  ○ Clean the hutch regularly
  ○ Use wire flooring (but there are serious implications for welfare and for the development of pododermatitis)

Prophylactic treatments
In many breeding colonies coccidiosis remains a serious problem despite reasonable levels of hygiene, and prophylactic treatment is necessary.
• Robenidine
  ○ Licensed (UK) in-feed anticoccidial, but only as an *aid* in the prevention of intestinal coccidiosis

- ○ Not effective against hepatic coccidia
- ○ Requires the animals to be fed primarily a pelleted diet, which may not be appropriate (see Nutritional requirements of rabbits, p. 105)
- Sulphonamides
  - ○ Can be used in the drinking water
  - ○ Risks emergence of resistant bacterial pathogens
  - ○ Perpetuates sulphonamide resistance among *Eimeria* strains
  - ○ Risks disturbing balance of caecal microflora

- Toltrazuril
  - ○ In-water preparation
  - ○ Useful agent for treatment of clinical coccidiosis, so use should perhaps be restricted to prevent development of resistant coccidia
  - ○ Higher risk of toxicity than other agents
- Amprolium
  - ○ Effective against both hepatic and intestinal forms
  - ○ Available in small volumes as an in-water medication (for pigeons)

ENCEPHALITOZOONOSIS

ENCEPHALITOZOON CUNICULI

- Intracellular microsporidian protozoon parasite
- Zoonotic to immunocompromised humans
  - ○ Primarily AIDS cases
  - ○ Diarrhoea, renal disease, keratoconjunctivitis
- Recognized for a long time as a renal infection in rabbit colonies
- Significance as cause of neurological disease in pet rabbits has only recently been realized

EPIDEMIOLOGY

- Prevalence of organism in healthy rabbit population at present unknown
  - ○ Wild rabbit populations generally 100% negative
  - ○ Amongst the UK domestic population, it is suspected that around 50% of clinically healthy rabbits may be seropositive
- Spores remain infective outside the host for up to 4 weeks

ROUTE

- Spores shed in urine
- Infective by ingestion or inhalation
- Ecto- and endoparasites may act as vectors/transport hosts

PATHOGENESIS

- Spore ingested or inhaled
- Infects host mucosal cell
- Multiplication within a vacuole within the host cell
- Reticuloendothelial system cells become infected and distribute organism around body
- Mature spores develop within vacuole
- Vacuole distends and cell ruptures releasing new spores into bloodstream (where they spread elsewhere in the body) or into urine (if renal cells rupture)
- Clinical disease is associated with the granulomatous inflammation which develops at the site of a ruptured cell (at which stage there may not be organisms present)

- Most commonly affected sites include:
  - Kidney
  - Brain
  - Spinal cord
  - Heart
  - Liver
  - The organisms can infect the lens of *in utero* kits

CLINICAL FINDINGS

Dependent on site affected.

CNS
- Various neurological problems
  - Head tilt
  - Paresis/paralysis
  - Tremors, seizures
  - Ataxia
  - Neurological urinary incontinence
  - Altered behaviour

Heart
- Myocarditis
- Dysrhythmia

Kidney
- Granulomatous nephritis
  - Usually subclinical but may contribute to CRF

Lens
- Cataract
- Localized or generalized phacoclastic uveitis

DIFFERENTIAL DIAGNOSIS

- Dependent on presenting clinical signs
- For 'head tilt' the most common differential is otitis interna/meningoencephalitis through spread of an upper respiratory tract infection

DIAGNOSIS

- Clinical signs and clinical examination (aim to rule out other possible causes)
- Haematology
- Encephalitozoon serology
  - Negative titre rules out *E. cuniculi*
  - Positive titre does *not* confirm *E. cuniculi* as the cause
- CSF analysis
  - Inflammatory changes are suggestive, but non-specific
- Urine analysis
  - Trichrome staining or PCR for *E. cuniculi* spores

THERAPY

- Anti-inflammatory treatments are most important in acute disease
  - Clinical signs are caused by granulomatous inflammation, *not* by presence of the organism
- Eradication of organism is possible by prolonged use of benzimidazoles
  - Length of course is chosen to prevent reinfestation
  - Fenbendazole at 20 mg/kg/day for 4 weeks

CONTROL

- Laboratory colonies are kept free of *E. cuniculi* by rigorous testing of all incoming stock and rejection of any animals serologically positive for *Encephalitozoon*
- As more becomes known about the incidence and significance of *Encephalitozoon* in the general population, routine use of benzimidazoles as a preventative measure may become indicated

HERPES SIMPLEX VIRUS INFECTION

EPIDEMIOLOGY

- Common viral infection of humans
  - Herpes labialis ('cold sores')
  - Herpetic stomatitis ('fever blisters')
- Anthropozoonosis
  - Spread from man to rabbit
  - Rabbit to rabbit spread is also common in laboratories
  - Potential for rabbit to human spread
    - Limited as most rabbit infection is not external
    - Keratitic cases could be infectious
- Rabbit used as laboratory model for herpes simplex virus investigation
- *In vitro* infection of rabbits easily achieved, yet clinical cases in pet rabbits are rarely reported
  - This may be due to poor recognition of signs and lack of post-mortem examination for histopathological confirmation
- Rabbit specific herpes viruses also occur
  - *Herpes cuniculi*
    - Subclinical infection in NZW
  - *Herpes sylvilagus*
    - Lymphoproliferative disease, myositis and pneumonia in cottontail rabbit species

ROUTE

- Unknown in few reported clinical cases, but suspected to be intranasal
- Experimentally virus is inoculated in various sites
  - Cornea, following light scarification
  - Intraocular
  - Intranasal or direct injection into the olfactory nerve

PATHOGENESIS

Local ocular infection after corneal inoculation
- Keratitis

Spread within nervous system
- Variable with inoculation site, with predictable patterns of distribution of microscopic lesions:
  - Corneal inoculation
    - Invades trigeminal nerve
    - Trigeminal ganglia used in experimental model to quantify viral penetration and replication after corneal inoculation
    - Spreads to brainstem, particularly cerebral hemispheres and ventral limbic system
  - Intraocular administration
    - Invades optic nerve
    - Spreads via optic chiasma to corpus geniculatum
  - Intranasal or olfactory nerve administration
    - Spread via olfactory nerve
    - Lesions in frontal and temporal lobes
- Few gross lesions
- Histopathological findings include:
  - Mild to moderate meningitis
  - Sharply demarcated areas of neuronal and glial necrosis within the cerebrum
  - Lymphocytic, plasma cell and histiocytic perivascular cuffing in the neuropil
  - Intranuclear basophilic or amphophilic inclusion bodies in glial cells and neurons, often filling the entire nucleus
- Can become latent infection, and be reactivated at a later stage

CLINICAL FINDINGS

- Restlessness
- Intermittent neurologic disturbances
  - Sudden running
  - Tonic–clonic spasm
  - Circling
  - Somersaulting
  - Seizures
  - Coma
  - Death

DIFFERENTIAL DIAGNOSIS

Any cause of acute onset neurological disturbance or seizure.

- Idiopathic
  - Epileptiform seizures with no apparent cause
  - Occasionally seen in rabbits
  - More prevalent in blue-eyed white breeds
- Encephalitozoonosis
  - Inflammatory response to encysted *Encephalitozoon* organisms can result in seizures either as a direct consequence of inflammation or as a consequence of restriction to bloodflow to other areas of the brain
  - Other parasitic infestations such as toxoplasmosis and aberrant ascarid migration may occasionally cause seizures
- Arteriosclerosis
  - Mineralization of meningeal blood vessels
  - Embolic incident
- Space occupying intracranial lesions
  - Abscessation (most commonly extension of an otitis)
  - Neoplasm

- Hypoxia
  - Severe cardiorespiratory disease
- Metabolic disease
  - End stages of renal or hepatic failure (especially hepatic lipidosis)
- End-stage systemic disease
  - Terminal stages of:
    — septicaemia
    — toxaemia (ingested toxins such as lead, or endotoxaemia)
    — VHD
- Cranial trauma

DIAGNOSIS

- Difficult to diagnose in live animal
- Clinical signs
- History of exposure to a human case
- Characteristic post-mortem findings
  - Histopathology
  - Immunohistochemical staining or PCR testing for confirmation

THERAPY

- No reports of successful therapy in naturally occurring cases
- Many reports of use of various antiviral drugs in experimental infections, e.g. aciclovir and famciclovir

CONTROL

- Avoid contact between humans with herpes labialis (cold sores) and herpetic stomatitis (fever blisters) and rabbits

LISTERIOSIS

EPIDEMIOLOGY

Listeria monocytogenes
- Rare
  - Small breeding units most susceptible
  - Rare in pets and in large colonies
- Immunosuppression usually a factor
  - Pregnancy
  - Poor nutrition
  - Concurrent disease

ROUTE

- Ingestion of contaminated feed

PATHOGENESIS

- Bacteraemic spread to uterus,
- Meningeal penetration

CLINICAL FINDINGS

- Abortion in breeding does, particularly in advanced pregnancy
- Metritis
- Signs of systemic infection – lethargy, inappetance, depression
- Sudden death
- Encephalitis with neurological signs (unusual)

POST-MORTEM FINDINGS

- Peritoneal fluid accumulation

- Fibrinous exudate on serosal surface of uterus
- Purulent metritis and dead fetuses in pregnant does
- Oedema of cervical and mesenteric lymph nodes
- Congestion and ecchymoses of viscera, particularly uterus
- Multiple pale miliary foci in liver and sometimes spleen
- Meningitis/encephalitis

DIFFERENTIAL DIAGNOSIS

- Pasteurellosis
- Septicaemia (yersiniosis)
- Encephalitozoonosis (neurological signs)

DIAGNOSIS

- Not usually possible in the individual animal
- Usually by culture of the organism post-mortem

THERAPY

- Antibiotics
  - Tetracyclines

CONTROL

- Routine husbandry and nutritional advice to avoid immunosuppression

INFECTIOUS DISEASES

MYXOMATOSIS

- Virus is an endemic subclinical poxvirus of *Sylvilagus* species of rabbits in South America
- Virus causes severe disease in aberrant domestic rabbit host (*Oryctolagus cuniculus*)
- Released illegally in France to control agricultural pest wild rabbits in 1952
- Spread across to UK in 1953 with widespread decimation of wild rabbit population

EPIDEMIOLOGY

- Different strains of virus and different portals of entry cause variable pathology
  - Different sizes and positions of 'myxomatous' growths
  - Different degrees of pulmonary oedema
  - Different extent of systemic involvement
- Currently infection waxes and wanes in the wild population as most rabbit populations have some immunity to the virus
- Most domestic rabbit outbreaks develop through direct or indirect contact with wild rabbits, rather than domestic–domestic spread
- Epidemiology varies with geographical locality due to the importance of various arthropod vectors

ROUTE

- Direct contact or close-range inhalation between rabbits in a colony
- Arthropod hosts
  - Especially rabbit fleas (*Spilopsyllus cuniculi*)
  - Also mosquitoes (*Aedes/Anopheles* spp.)
  - Cat/dog fleas (*Ctenocephalides* spp.)
  - *Cheyletiella*

- Rabbit fleas may be introduced to an 'isolated' domestic rabbit through 'hitchhiker' fleas on predators such as domestic cats or foxes
- Calypterid flies (*Musca*, *Calliphora*, *Lucilia*, etc.) are less of a concern as they do not provide an intradermal inoculation of the virus

PATHOGENESIS

- Sequential replication at the infection site and regional lymph node
- Typically, skin lesion 4 days post inoculation enlarges to 3 cm at 10 days post inoculation
- Cell-associated viraemia leads to generalized infection with replication within lymphoid system
- Eyelid swelling and secondary conjunctivitis by day 9
- Swollen and purulent lesions develop on mucocutaneous junctions and earbases
- Virulent disease in farmed colonies leads to inhaled spread and primary pulmonary site of infection, with pneumonia and secondary pasteurellosis at 7–20 days instead of skin masses

CLINICAL FINDINGS

- Skin masses
- Rhinitis, conjunctivitis, pneumonia
- Lesions of lips, nares, eyelids, genitalia
- Lethargy, pyrexia

DIFFERENTIAL DIAGNOSIS

- Pasteurellosis (respiratory/conjunctival signs)
- Syphilis (genital signs)

DIAGNOSIS

- Colony history, vaccination history
- Clinical signs
- Progression
- Parasitology
  - Presence of *Psilopsyllus cuniculi* on a domestic rabbit would be highly suggestive of positive diagnosis

THERAPY

- Prognosis is very poor in systemically affected rabbits
- Consider quality of life/welfare/euthanasia at the outset

Many clinical signs and causes of fatality are due to secondary bacterial infections, inanition and dehydration (due to inability to see and lethargy) and in wild rabbits predation. Aggressive antibiosis, fluid therapy, NSAIDs, supportive feeding and general nursing may control the disease long enough for immune response and viral clearance in some rabbits, but this depends on host immune status and virulence of the viral strain involved, and some cases will survive for several weeks before finally developing renal failure.

- Maintaining the rabbit at 29.4°C has been shown to increase survival rate

CONTROL

- Prevention/control of insect vectors
  - Prevention of contact with wild rabbits
  - Flea control
  - Mosquito netting over hutch front
  - Ultraviolet fly killers (as used in catering establishments) in colony housing

Vaccination

- Generally poor immune response to killed pox virus vaccines
- Attenuated myxomavirus strains effective in some studies, but problems with virulence vs. host immunity
- Shope-fibroma virus
  - Similar pox virus endemic in a different wild *Sylvilagus* species of rabbit (*Sylvilagus floridanus*)
  - Stimulates cross immunity to *Myxomavirus*
  - Wild strain shope-fibroma virus causes fibromas at the inoculation site which persist for 3–12 weeks
    - Domestic rabbits in areas of the USA with a wild *Sylvilagus floridanus* population and abundant insect vectors may develop this as a multifocal disease due to multiple bites by mosquitoes
  - Attenuated shope-fibromavirus vaccine available in the UK provides 6–10 months duration of immunity
- Essential that 0.1 ml of the vaccine is given intradermally
- Base vaccination protocol on local endemic status
  - If local high risk of myxomatosis vaccinate every 6–8 months
  - If no obvious local myxomatosis risk, possibly just vaccinate annually in springtime to cover main risk periods

INFECTIOUS DISEASES

PASTEURELLOSIS

EPIDEMIOLOGY

- Many strains with variable pathogenicity
- In pet rabbits usually *not* a primary pathogen, but an opportunist or secondary pathogen
- Can act as primary pathogen in colony situations

Factors predisposing to clinical Pasteurellosis include:
- Inhaled irritants
  ○ Ammonia
  ○ Petroleum
  ○ Air fresheners
  ○ Disinfectants
- Co-infection with cytotoxic *Bordetella bronchiseptica*
- Corticosteroid use or stress
- Cachexia
  ○ Dental disease
- Myxomatosis
- Pulmonary neoplasia
- Pregnancy/parturition/lactation
- Overcrowding
- Genetic predisposition
  ○ Chinchilla more susceptible than Blue Beveren

ROUTE

- Direct (nose to nose) contact
- Airborne spread
- Fomites/contaminated water supplies

PATHOGENESIS

- Spread to newborn rabbits shortly after birth by nuzzling of dam
  ○ During parturition if vaginal infection
- Pre-weaning kits protected by maternally-derived antibodies
- Colonization/subclinical infection of nares

- Incubation period in clinical outbreaks of 8 days to 3 weeks
- Abundant in nasal mucus, though absent from sinuses
- Normally mucociliary clearance balances bacterial proliferation until IgA and cell-mediated immune response develops, when either bacteriological clearance, or nares or tympanic bulla carrier status follows
- Clinical disease because of decreased mucociliary clearance or decreased cellular or humoral immunity
- Infection progresses from nares through rest of respiratory tract and tympanic bullae

CLINICAL FINDINGS

- Variable
  ○ Acute
  ○ Subacute
  ○ Chronic
  ○ Subclinical
- Purulent rhinitis
  ○ 'Snuffles'
  ○ Nose often 'wiped' leading to presentation with clear nose but matted hair on inner aspect of carpi
  ○ Chronic infections, especially co-infections with *Bordetella*, lead to atrophic rhinitis as a result of local toxin release
- Conjunctivitis
- Pneumonia
  ○ Toxins released by *Pasteurella* can induce inflammatory changes of pneumonia even in the absence of infection within the lungs
  ○ Subclinical pneumonia +/− chronic pulmonary abscessation are common in apparently healthy rabbits
- Tracheitis

- Dacryocystitis
  - Usually primarily an obstructive disease due to incisor root elongation
  - *Pasteurella* colonizes because of decreased clearance caused by the obstruction
- Otitis media
  - Often not clinical
  - Common incidental finding at post-mortem examination or on radiographs
  - Clinical vestibular disease is usually a consequence of spread of infection to otitis interna or to brainstem
- Abscesses
  - (Perioral abscessation and abscesses of bite wounds are often not *Pasteurella* but anaerobic infections)
- Metritis
  - Infertility in breeding colonies
- Septicaemia

DIFFERENTIAL DIAGNOSIS

Respiratory
- Bordetellosis
  - Usually serous only
  - Common copathogen with *Pasteurella*
- *Staphylococcus* or *Pseudomonas* infection
- Nasal foreign body
- Myxomatosis
- Pulmonary or nasal neoplasia

Abscesses
- Anaerobes
- *Staphylococcus*

Genital infection
- Cystic endometrial hyperplasia
- Uterine adenocarcinoma
- Syphilis

Look for underlying factors even if *Pasteurella* is confirmed.

DIAGNOSIS

- Identification of underlying factors
- Colony history of disease
- Various diagnostic imaging and biopsy techniques to identify extent of lesions and to rule out concurrent neoplastic or viral disease

Bacteriological culture and sensitivity
- Test of choice in clinically affected pet animals
  - Usual test (repeated several times over 4 weeks) used when developing 'Pasteurella-free' laboratory colonies
- 'Pus' is usually sterile neutrophil debris
- Needs to be deep swab from mucosa 1–3 cm inside nasal cavity; usually some epistaxis
- Risk of missing infection if pockets are within tympanic bullae or nasal sinuses
- Many *Pasteurella* strains are temperature-sensitive and have peculiar culture medium requirements, so are not easily isolated in clinical practice

Serological testing
- Seroconversion (IgG) only with chronic infections
- Positive titre suggests prior exposure and possible, but not definite, carrier status
- Rising titre on paired sera suggests recent or active infection
- Negative titre does not completely rule out *Pasteurella*-associated disease

PCR testing
- Not widely available at present
- Combination of serology and PCR gives superior results to culture

THERAPY

- Identify and, where possible, eliminate all underlying factors

- Systemic antibiosis
  - Tetracyclines
  - (Penicillins, chloramphenicol – good effect vs. *Pasteurella* but potential toxicity)
  - Fluoroquinolones
  - (Cephalosporins; gentamycin; azithromycin – potential toxicity)
  - Potentiated sulphonamides
- Local treatment
  - Intranasal antibiotics
  - Nebulized antibiotics and mucolytics
- Supportive care
  - Severe cases may be unable to eat/drink, leading to cachexia and dehydration

CONTROL

- Prevention of underlying factors through appropriate husbandry and nutrition

- Isolation, screening bacteriology and barrier housing of 'Pasteurella-free' colonies

Vaccination

- Clinical disease is usually a result of impaired function of an already activated cell mediated immune system, so vaccination is unlikely to be effective
  - Even *in vitro*, serum with confirmed anti-*Pasteurella* IgG is not bactericidal
- Injectable vaccines are ineffective because circulating antibody (IgG) is not protective on mucosal surface
  - Experimental intranasal vaccines beneficial against the same pathogenic strain and serotype, but not completely protective against colonization; not good cross reaction between serotypes; limited availability
  - No evidence that injectable sheep *Pasteurella* vaccine has any beneficial effect

TOXOPLASMOSIS

EPIDEMIOLOGY

- The rabbit, together with most mammals, is an end stage host for *Toxoplasma gondii*
- Rabbits are generally resistant to clinical effects
  - Causes severe fatal disease of some hares
- Clinical toxoplasmosis is rare in domestic pets
- Zoonotic, but only by handling or eating undercooked rabbit meat
  - Wild rabbits may constitute an important reservoir for infection of naive cats

PATHOGENESIS

- Primarily an enteric parasite of cats
- In non-felid species, oocysts hatch in the duodenum, enter the bloodstream and pass to various sites in the body
- 'Cysts' are established within infected tissues; they are often asymptomatic and remain for the lifespan of the rabbit
- Rabbits do not shed infective oocysts in their faeces
- Young or immune compromised individuals are most susceptible to clinical disease
- Pregnant and nursing does in colonies are particularly affected

ROUTE

- Ingestion of food contaminated with faeces of an infected (and shedding) cat

CLINICAL FINDINGS

Two presentations:
- Acute systemic disease

- ○ Anorexia
- ○ Pyrexia
- ○ Lethargy
- ○ May be hepatosplenomegaly, with spleen 10× normal size
- ○ Death after a few days
- CNS disease
  - ○ Posterior paralysis
  - ○ Muscle tremors
  - ○ Seizures

DIAGNOSIS

- Difficult
  - ○ Definitive diagnosis is usually post mortem
- Cytology of impression smears or histopathology
- Samples need to be taken from a fresh (less than a few hours) carcass or the organism becomes unidentifiable

DIFFERENTIAL DIAGNOSIS

- Various causes of acute lethargy/pyrexia
  - ○ (Pasteurellosis, yersiniosis)
- Various causes of CNS disturbance
  - ○ (Encephalitozoonosis, pasteurellosis)

THERAPY

- Potentiated sulphonamides

CONTROL

- Avoid access to grazing or stored feed that has been contaminated with cat faeces
- Wash all fresh vegetables before feeding

TREPONEMIASIS (SYPHILIS)

EPIDEMIOLOGY

Treponema paraluis-cuniculi
- Spirochaete infection
  - ○ Non-zoonotic
- Causes a disease referred to as 'rabbit syphilis' or 'vent disease'
- Common in some breeding colonies
  - ○ Asymptomatic carriers are common, and perpetuate the infection within an affected colony
    - – Does that have had six litters, and bucks that have been in a breeding programme for over 12 months are highly likely to be seropositive
  - ○ Difficult to pinpoint source of infection within colony because of asymptomatic carrier status and long incubation period – may have been brought in with new stock many months before

ROUTE

- Venereal
- Vertically at parturition and lactation

PATHOGENESIS

- Readily transmitted during mating
- Long incubation period (10–16 weeks)
- Lesions first appear as reddened areas of perineum/genitalia
- These progress to oedema, vesicles 1–2 mm in diameter, ulceration and scabbing
  - ○ At this stage they can be painful and inhibit mating, causing a reduced conception rate
- Grooming activity by the animal leads to infection elsewhere, e.g. lips, nose, eyelids

INFECTIOUS DISEASES

- ○ These lesions tend to be proliferative and scaly and can be misdiagnosed as dermatophytosis, myxomatosis or parasitic lesions
- Inguinal lymph nodes may become enlarged
- Vesicles coalesce and burst and develop into crusting lesions
- Infected colonies have increased incidence of metritis, placental retention and neonatal deaths
- Clinical disease is generally self limiting
  - ○ Immune competent individuals may show little or no clinically evident disease when first infected, but remain asymptomatic carriers
  - ○ Disease may recrudesce when the animal is stressed or has concurrent illness

CLINICAL FINDINGS

- Reddening, oedema, vesicles, ulceration and scabbing of mucocutaneous junctions, particularly genitalia, but also face
  - ○ Forepaws and ears also occasionally affected
- Reduced reproductive performance in a breeding colony (decreased fertility, increased metritis, abortion)
- Bucks which have recovered from the clinically evident infection (but which are therefore likely to be asymptomatic carriers) often have a characteristic star shaped scrotal scar

DIFFERENTIAL DIAGNOSIS

- Individual animals
  - ○ Dermatophytosis
  - ○ Parasitic infestation, e.g. *Psoroptes cuniculi*; *Notoedres* or *Sarcoptes* in endemic areas
  - ○ Anal papilloma

- Multiple animals in a group
  - ○ Mild strains of myxomatosis
- If facial lesions only
  - ○ Burns (heat, electrical, caustic) to lips
  - ○ Trauma from biting bars of cage

DIAGNOSIS

- Presumptive diagnosis often possible on clinical signs alone, especially in group outbreaks
- Confirmatory tests
  - ○ Dark field microscopy if available
  - ○ Histopathology (requires silver stains, so discuss with laboratory before submission)
  - ○ Serological tests
    - — Reliable cross reaction with *Treponema pallidum* using human syphilis tests
    - — Up to 25% of clinically healthy rabbits are seropositive

THERAPY

- Penicillins
  - ○ Classical reports centre on injections of penicillins given 7–21 days apart
  - ○ Penicillin is treatment of choice in humans, and when initial reports of treatment were made few other antibiotics were available
  - ○ Allows treatment of whole colony on same dates with only single handling each dose, so easy management in large colony
  - ○ Risks of penicillins causing enterotoxaemia
- Tetracyclines
  - ○ Treatment of choice in penicillin-sensitive humans
  - ○ Tetracyclines are far safer for rabbits but require a more intensive therapeutic regime

— Injections of long-acting oxytetra-cycline every 3 days
— Oral administration once or twice a day for several weeks
○ Difficult in colony situations where rabbits are not used to being handled and twice-daily oral administration is not possible for management reasons
○ A far safer option for treatment of small colonies and pet animals

Other agents could also be considered including chloramphenicol, and related antibiotics, tiamulin and cephalexin. Fluoroquinolones have variable activity against *Treponema* spp. and may suppress the clinical signs but not eliminate the organism.

CONTROL

• Routine monthly inspection of breeding stock
  ○ Especially if signs of decreased fertility
  ○ Eversion of vulva or prepuce to examine for lesions or pus
• Examination of the scrotum of breeding bucks before introduction to the colony
  ○ Ideally, quarantine would be applied, but the incubation period of several months makes this impractical
• Serological testing or prophylactic antibiotic treatment of potential introductions to a breeding colony

TULARAEMIA

EPIDEMIOLOGY

Francisella tularensis
• Common in wild rabbits in the USA
• Rare in *Oryctolagus*, especially in domestic rabbits
• Zoonotic

ROUTE

• Insect transmission or direct contact
  ○ Particularly through bites

PATHOGENESIS

• Invades conjunctiva or directly implanted into skin via bites by host or insect vector

CLINICAL FINDINGS

• Acute septicaemic disease

DIFFERENTIAL DIAGNOSIS

• Other forms of septicaemia and viraemia

DIAGNOSIS

• Post-mortem only
• Most likely as a result of investigation into rare zoonotic disease cases

INFECTIOUS DISEASES

TYZZER'S DISEASE

EPIDEMIOLOGY

Clostridium piliformis
- Formerly classified *Bacillus piliformis*
- Uncommon in pet rabbits
- Can affect any age
- Affects many rodent species
  - Wild rodent reservoir of infection
- Most clinical cases involve immuno-compromised animals

ROUTE

- Ingestion of food contaminated by the organism

PATHOGENESIS

- Organism ingested and infects intestinal and caecal cells
  - Obligate intracellular organism
- Immunocompetent animals may develop subclinical carrier status
- Immunocompromise triggers disease

In acute stages
- Enteritis
- Intestinal oedema
- Bacteraemic spread and can affect myocardium causing sudden death

Surviving animals develop chronic stages
- Small intestinal fibrosis and stenosis
- Necrotic hepatitis

CLINICAL FINDINGS

Young rabbits
- Acute watery diarrhoea
- Dehydration
- Depression
- Death

Older animals
- Chronic diarrhoea
- Weight loss

DIFFERENTIAL DIAGNOSIS

- Acute
  - Colibacillosis
  - Coccidiosis
- Chronic
  - Many differentials of chronic weight loss

DIAGNOSIS

- Difficult in individual animal
- Not usually made in acute cases
- Intestinal biopsy may confirm fibrosis in chronic weight loss cases
  - Causative organism not present at this stage
- In colonies, post-mortem examination of affected animals is indicated
  - Focal hepatic necrosis < 2 mm in diameter (less common than in rodents)
  - Necrotic areas of GIT (especially caecum and proximal colon) and myocardium
  - Oedema of GIT, particularly caecal wall
  - Histopathological examination of lesions using silver stains to identify intracellular organism
  - Organism cannot be cultured on standard media, but tissue culture methods are available
- Serological testing

THERAPY

- Antibiosis
  - Tetracyclines
  - Prolonged courses to avoid reinfection from environmental spores
- Supportive therapy
  - Fluids
  - Supplemental nutrition
  - Stress reduction
- Prognosis poor even if infection controlled
  - Due to fibrotic changes in intestines
- In a colony, culling of affected animals is indicated to reduce environmental contamination and exposure of healthy stock

CONTROL

- Routine husbandry and nutritional advice to avoid immunocompromise
  - Stress reduction, environmental enrichment
- Avoid rodent access to rabbit housing and food (including hay) stores
  - (Spores are resistant and persist for a long time on foodstuffs after the source of infection is removed)
- Bleach (3% sodium hypochlorite) is effective, even against spores

YERSINIOSIS

(Pseudotuberculosis, rodentosis)

EPIDEMIOLOGY

Yersinia pseudotuberculosis
- Common infection of rodents
  - Particularly cavies (guinea pigs)
  - Also some aviary birds (passerines, touracos)
- Moderately common in wild rabbits
- Rare in domestic pets

ROUTE

- Ingestion of infected faeces or urine of wild rodents and birds through contamination of food

PATHOGENESIS

- Organism multiplies in intestine and invades lymphoid tissue of GIT
- Haematogenous spread to the spleen (and septicaemia)

CLINICAL FINDINGS

- Non-specific
  - Lethargy
  - Cachexia
  - Occasionally diarrhoea
  - Weight loss

DIFFERENTIAL DIAGNOSIS

- Any systemic disease causing lethargy

DIAGNOSIS

- Definitive diagnosis difficult in the live rabbit
  - Haematology may reveal changes in leucocyte numbers and morphology suggestive of bacterial infection
  - Abdominal palpation may reveal a large spleen or nodular swelling of the liver
- Post-mortem examination
  - Spleen is enlarged and has multiple necrotic foci on the surface
  - Similar lesions in the liver

- Foci also at ileocaecal ampulla and other intestinal lymphoid aggregates
- Advanced cases have caseous necrosis of mesenteric lymph nodes

THERAPY

- Prolonged courses of antibiotics (several weeks) to affected and contact animals

- Fluoroquinolones
- Tetracyclines

CONTROL

- Exclude rodents and wild birds from the rabbit's housing and food stores
- Wash all fresh vegetables before feeding to rabbits

SECTION 5
THERAPEUTICS

INTRODUCTION

With the exception of certain antibacterial agents which can have severe adverse effects through alteration of the caecal microflora, and drugs which reduce intestinal motility, rabbits are generally resistant to drug intoxication. There are, however, major differences in pharmacological parameters such as drug uptake from the gastrointestinal tract and rates of metabolism and excretion. Other parameters may play effects, such as drug metabolism by intestinal microorganisms and drug recycling through ingestion of caecotrophs. Although many texts concerning diseases of farmed or laboratory rabbits discuss medication of the animals by inclusion of therapeutic agents in the feed or in the drinking water, these routes are not appropriate for domestic pets as the actual intake of a single individual rabbit cannot be guaranteed. In particular, many medications will reduce the palatability of drinking water, resulting in both insufficient intake of the drug and also dehydration. It should be noted that few of the drugs discussed below are licensed in the UK for use in rabbits: attention must be paid to the prescribing 'cascade', and also to restrictions on the use of drugs in food-animal species.

ANTIMICROBIALS

FLUOROQUINOLONES

Enrofloxacin available as a licensed preparation for rabbits in the UK.
- Good oral bioavailability
- Wide tissue distribution, including CSF
- Action
  - Boad-spectrum antibacterials
  - Particular effect against many of the bacteria responsible for disease in rabbits, such as *Pasteurella*, *Bordetella*, *Staphylococcus* and the rarer *Listeria* and *Yersinia*
  - No effect against anaerobic bacteria, so not a good choice for bite wounds and tooth related abscesses
- Toxicity
  - Arthropathy in juveniles
  - Blindness has been reported in other species
  - Some rabbits become inappetent or develop transient mild diarrhoea
- Dose
  - Enrofloxacin 10 mg/kg PO q12 h.

CHLORAMPHENICOL

- Poor oral bioavailability
- Restrictions on use, especially since the rabbit is a food-animal species
- Related drugs such as fluorphenicol may have some uses
- Action
  - Broad-spectrum, bacteriostatic
  - Good penetration, widely and rapidly distributed
- Toxicity
  - Dose-dependent bone marrow suppression usually reversible on drug withdrawal
- Dose
  - 30 mg/kg IM q24 h

TETRACYCLINES

When given orally, tetracyclines may chelate calcium, potentially restricting absorption of both the therapeutic drug and calcium itself. Do not administer the drug at the same time as calcium-containing supplementation.

THERAPEUTICS

- Action
  - Broad spectrum
  - Includes good activity against *Pasteurella*
  - Also active against a range of anaerobes
  - Good tissue penetration including bones and teeth
- Toxicity
  - Rare
  - Anorexia at extremely high doses
  - Decreased water intake and poor absorption when given in the drinking water
- Doses
  - Oxytetracycline 50 mg/kg PO q12 h
  - Oxytetracycline 30 mg/kg IM (long-acting preparation) every 3 days
  - Doxycycline 4 mg/kg q12–24 h

POTENTIATED SULPHONAMIDES

Available as a palatable human paediatric suspension in the UK.
- Action
  - Broad spectrum, including some anaerobes; bactericidal
  - Inactivated in the presence of exudates and debris, limiting their effect against established abscesses
- Toxicity
  - Rare
  - Renal damage seen in carnivores does not occur because of the naturally alkaline urine of the rabbit
- Doses
  - Trimethoprim/sulphadiazine 48 mg/kg SC q24 h
  - Trimethoprim/sulphamethoxazole (Septrin paediatric) and other oral preparations 30 mg/kg PO q12 h
  - Silver sulphadiazine topically as necessary, e.g. to marsupialized abscesses

PENICILLINS

High risk of potentially fatal dysenterobiosis (antibiotic related enterotoxaemia), especially with oral administration.
Ampicillin seems a particularly high risk
- Action
  - Bactericidal
  - Broad spectrum, including anaerobes
  - May be useful in abscess cases where safer antibiotics have already failed
- Dose
  - Procaine +/– benzocaine penicillin 40 mg/kg (40 000 u/kg) SC
- For *Treponema cuniculi* (consider the use of safer drugs such as doxycycline) 80 mg/kg procaine penicillin once a week for 3–6 weeks

CEPHALOSPORINS

Moderate risk of dysenterobiosis (antibiotic related enterotoxaemia), especially with oral administration. Less risk than with penicillins. Cephalexin appears to be reasonably safe.
- Action
  - Broad spectrum antibiosis
  - Includes anaerobes
  - Good tissue penetration, including bone
- Toxicity
  - Dysenterobiosis, diarrhoea, anorexia
- Suggested doses
  - Cephalexin 15–30 mg/kg SC q24 h
  - Cephalexin 15 mg/kg PO q12 h

AMINOGLYCOSIDES

No GI absorption; poor CNS penetration; need multiple injections each day to maintain therapeutic levels; risks of nephrotoxicity.

THERAPEUTICS

May be useful in management of severe systemic infection, and may be of use by local injection into abscess capsule.

Licensed ocular preparation in the UK.
- Action
  - Broad spectrum, bacteriostatic
- Doses
  - Amikacin or gentamicin 2 mg/kg IM/IV q6 h with supplemental fluid therapy

MACROLIDES, LINCOSAMIDES AND AZALIDES

Macrolides (e.g. erythromycin) and lincosamides (lincomycin, clindamycin) carry a severe risk of inducing fatal dysenterobiosis (antibiotic related enterotoxaemia). Use of these drugs is restricted in rabbits to local implantation of capsules (Antirobe) or antibiotic impregnated methylmethacrylate beads into abscess sites.

Other macrolides such as tylosin and tilmycosin have been used in attempt to develop single dose or weekly dose protocols for elimination of *Pasteurella* from colonies. These protocols have been developed in situations where adverse effects in a small number of rabbits would not necessarily be a problem. Fatal adverse reactions and dysenterobiosis problems are possible, and so these protocols are not appropriate for single pet rabbits.
- Azithromycin (an azalide)
  - Shows promise because of a very broad spectrum of activity
  - Includes many anaerobes
  - Excellent penetration into tissues, including bone
  - Safer than other drugs in this group
- Dose
  - Azithromycin 25 mg/kg PO q24 h

METRONIDAZOLE

Liquid formulations available, though many rabbits do not like the 'cherry' flavour. Tablets have very bitter taste.
- Action restricted to effect against anaerobic bacteria, but very good effects against these
- Toxicity
  - Neurotoxicity in other species
- Dose
  - Metronidazole 20 mg/kg PO q12 h

ANTIPARASITIC AGENTS

BENZIMIDAZOLES

Many preparations are available, predominantly developed as anthelmintics.
- Action
  - Effective against many roundworms and tapeworms.
  - Also effective against some protozoa; notably, from rabbit perspective, effective against *Encephalitozoon cuniculi*. Although other drugs have been investigated, fenbendazole is at present the only drug with published data supporting *in vivo* effects against *E. cuniculi*.
- Toxicity
  - Bone marrow suppression (reduced WBC counts) is possible but adverse effects not widely reported.
- Doses
  - As an anthelmintic 20 mg/kg PO q24 h for 5 days
  - Against *E. cuniculi* 20 mg/kg PO q24 h for 4 weeks

THERAPEUTICS

AVERMECTINS

- Primarily used in rabbits against ectoparasites, as limited effectiveness against *Passalurus*
- Dose
  - Ivermectin 200 to 400 μg/kg PO/SC/ percutaneous, repeated after 10 to 14 days
  - Selamectin 12 mg/kg percutaneously

SULPHONAMIDES

- Effective against coccidia, though with variable and increasing resistance
- Sulphaquinoxaline is the most effective
- Doses
  - Trimethoprim/sulphamethoxazole 30 mg/kg PO q24 h
  - Sulphaquinoxaline 1–3 mg/litre of drinking water
  - Sulphadimidine 100–233 mg/litre of drinking water
  - Sulphadimidine 100 mg/kg PO q24 h

AMPROLIUM

- Useful in water treatment for anticoccidial prophylaxis
- Dose
  - Amprolium 2.3 ml of 3.84% solution per litre of drinking water

ROBENIDINE

Licensed in the UK for in-feed use as an aid to prevention of coccidiosis.
- Dose 50–66 g/tonne of pellets

TOLTRAZURIL

- Highly effective anticoccidial treatment
- Greater potential for toxic effects than other prophylactic agents
- Dose
  - 25 mg/kg PO daily for 2 days, repeated after a 5 day break

SEDATIVES, ANALGESICS AND ANTI-INFLAMMATORY AGENTS

Sedatives mentioned below are those of use for light to moderate sedation and anxiolytic effects to allow clinical examination, blood sampling and stress free hospitalization of rabbits. A full discussion of anaesthesia is beyond the scope of this text.

OPIOIDS AND COMBINATIONS

- Analgesia with mild to profound sedation depending on agent and dose
- Fentanyl–fluanisone may be available as a licensed preparation for rabbits in the

UK, and is a moderate sedative with excellent analgesic properties
- Sedation may be reversable by use of a partial agonist with less sedative effects whilst still maintaining some analgesia
- Adverse effects of concern include gastrointestinal, respiratory and cardiovascular depression
- Doses
  - Butorphanol 0.1–0.4 mg/kg SC/IM/ IV (lasts only 2–4 hours)
  - Buprenorphine 0.01–0.05 mg/kg IV/SC q6–q12 h
  - Fentanyl–fluanisone 0.2 ml/kg IM

THERAPEUTICS

BENZODIAZEPINES

- Sedation, anxiolytic effects, muscle relaxation
- May provide some degree of appetite stimulation
- Negligible adverse cardiovascular or GI effects
- No analgesic properties
- Dose
  - Midazolam 0.5–2 mg/kg IM/IV as necessary
  - Diazepam 1–2 mg/kg IM/IV as necessary

NON-STEROIDAL ANTI-INFLAMMATORY DRUGS (NSAIDS)

- Generally appear well tolerated in rabbits
- Potential for gastric ulceration or renal impairment as adverse effects
- Doses
  - Carprofen 2–4 mg/kg PO/SC q24 h
  - Meloxicam 0.1–0.2 mg/kg PO q24 h
  - Ketoprofen 1–3 mg/kg PO q12 h

CORTICOSTEROIDS

There are few indications for the use of corticosteroids in rabbits. Rabbits are particularly prone to stress related disorders, and in particular corticosteroids can have adverse effects on gut motility and predispose to gastric ulceration. Many rabbits are subclinically infected with organisms such as *Pasteurella multocida*, *Encephalitozoon cuniculi* and *Clostridia* spp., and the use of corticosteroids may allow these conditions to progress to clinical disease. The main indications for corticosteroid use are as a single IV bolus of a soluble preparation for shock or acute inflammatory diseases (especially encephalitozoonosis). Allergic and autoimmune diseases are not widely reported in rabbits, but may occur. Corticosteroids may be used as part of the management of neoplastic, and particularly lymphoproliferative, disorders. Non-specific pain or inflammation should be treated with NSAIDs rather than corticosteroids.

- Dose
  - Prednisolone 0.5–2 mg/kg PO/SC
  - Dexamethasone 1–2 mg/kg IM/IV

GASTROINTESTINAL DRUGS

MOTILITY MODIFYING AGENTS

Buscopan
Possibly indicated in cases of gut spasm or hypermotility, but contraindicated in cases of hypomotility which is the usual situation in rabbit GI disease.

Metoclopramide
Central and local prokinetic and anti-emetic. *In vitro* is effective on adult small intestine smooth muscle cells, but not neonatal cells.

- Action
  - Promotes gastric emptying and intestinal motility
  - May be of benefit in palliation of 'head tilt' cases which may have central nausea
- Toxicity
  - Rare
  - Contraindicated in cases of physical GI obstruction
- Dose
  - Metoclopramide 0.5 mg/kg SC/PO q6–q12 h

THERAPEUTICS

Cisapride
- Action
  - Locally active prokinetic agent
  - Promotes gastric emptying, increases small intestine and colonic motility, stimulates appetite
  - *In vitro* evidence suggests cisapride has effects on neonatal intestinal muscle (cf. metoclopramide)
- Toxicity
  - Rare in rabbits, though potential for drug interactions and for teratogenic effects
  - Contraindicated in cases of physical GI obstruction
- Dose
  - Cisapride 0.5 mg/kg PO q6–q12 h

Human fatalities following cisapride use have led to cessation of production, with cisapride available at the time of writing only on direct prescription from the manufacturers on a named patient basis. This drug is likely to become unavailable in the near future, and though there are drugs with similar action being developed there is little data available on the suitability of these agents for use in rabbits.

ANTI-ULCER TREATMENTS

Omeprazole
- Inhibits gastric acid production by parietal cells
- Experimentally shown to decrease gastric ulcer formation in indomethacin treated rabbits, and to markedly elevate post-prandial gastric pH

- Dose difficult to administer as only available as large capsules

H₂ antagonists
- Reduce gastric acid secretion and pepsin output, thereby reducing two possible factors in gastric ulceration
- May stimulate gut motility
- Dose
  - Ranitidine 2 mg/kg IV q24 h; 2–5 mg/kg PO q12 h

VERAPAMIL

Calcium channel blocker, mainly used in other species for cardiac arrhythmias.
- Inhibits post-operative adhesion formation
- Dose
  - Verapamil 200 µg/kg SC three times daily for a total of nine doses

CHOLESTYRAMINE

- Action
  - Ion exchange resin
  - Increases rate of cholesterol metabolism by removing products of metabolism (bile acids) from the gut before reabsorbtion
  - Also binds fat soluble and bacterial toxins
  - Used as a preventative/treatment agent in rabbits at risk of enterotoxaemia
- Dose
  - 0.5 g/kg PO/on food q12 h

REPRODUCTIVE TREATMENTS

BUSERELIN

UK licensed product for induction of ovulation for reproductive manipulation (improvement of conception rates) and artificial insemination.
- FSH/LH analogue
- Dose
  - 0.2 ml Receptal® per rabbit SC

PROLIGESTONE

- Progesterone analogue

- Of short term use in control of pseudo-pregnancy signs
- Dose
  - 30 mg/kg SC injection

CABERGOLINE

- Prolactin inhibitor
- Useful for short term suppression of lactation (e.g. in false pregnancy or mastitis)
- Dose
  - 5 µg/kg q24 h for 4–6 days

MISCELLANEOUS TREATMENTS

EDTA (SODIUM CALCIUM EDETATE) AND PENICILLAMINE

- Chelating agents for heavy metals, particularly lead
- Dose
  - EDTA 13–27.5 mg/kg SC/IV q6 h for 5 days
  - Penicillamine 30 mg/kg PO q12 h

NANDROLONE

- Anabolic steroid
- Inhibits catabolic changes, promotes increase of muscle mass, promotes RBC regeneration
- Appetite stimulant
- Dose
  - Nandrolone 2 mg/kg IM/SC

THERAPEUTICS

BIBLIOGRAPHY

Anon. (1999) Green light for greens. *Rabbiting On*, Winter. Rabbit Welfare Association, Horsham.

Ashton, N., Cook, C. & Clegg, F. (1976) Encephalitozoonosis (nosematosis) causing bilateral cataract in a rabbit. *British Journal of Ophthalmology*, 60, 618–31.

Besch-Williford, C. (1997) Tyzzer's disease in rabbits. In: *Rabbit Medicine and Procedures for Practitioners*. Program and Abstracts, House Rabbit Society Veterinary Conference, Berkeley, CA.

Bodeker, D., Turck, O., Loven, E., Weiberneit, D. & Wegner, W. (1995) Pathophysiological and functional aspects of the megacolon-syndrome of homozygous spotted rabbits. *Journal of the Veterinary Medical Association*, 42, 549–59.

Boorman, G.A. & Bree, M.M. (1969) Diabetes insipidus syndrome in a rabbit. *Journal of the American Veterinary Medical Association*, 155, 1218–20.

Boot, R., Thuis, H. & Wieten, G. (1985) Multifactorial analysis of antimicrobial sensitivity of *Bordatella bronchiseptica* isolates from guinea pigs, rabbits and rats. *Laboratory Animals*, 29, 45–9.

Boydell, P. (2000) Nervous system and disorders. In: Flecknell, P (Ed.), *BSAVA Manual of Rabbit Medicine and Surgery*. British Small Animal Veterinary Association, Quedgeley, pp. 57–61.

Brooks, D. (2004) Nutrition and gastrointestinal physiology. In: Quesenberry, K.E. & Carpenter, J.W. (Eds), *Ferrets, Rabbits and Rodents: Clinical Medicine and Surgery* (2nd Edn). W.B. Saunders, Philadelphia, pp. 155–60.

Brown, S. (2001) Head tilt and other neurological disease in the house rabbit. *Small Mammal Health Series*. (http://www.veterinarypartner.com/Content.plx?P=A&A=485&S=5&SourceID=43) Accessed 12/11/04.

Brown, S. (2001) Hind limb weakness in the rabbit. *Small Mammal Health Series*. (http://www.veterinarypartner.com/Content.plx?P=A&C=10&A=490&S=0) Accessed 12/11/04.

Brown, S. (2004) Organomegaly. In: Meredith, A. (Ed.), *CD-Lapis*. Vetstream, Winchester.

Capello, V. (2004) Diagnosis and treatment of urolithiasis in pet rabbits. *Exotic DVM*, 6(2), 15–22.

Capucci, L., Nardin, A. & Lavazza, A. (1997) Seroconversion in an industrial unit of rabbits infected with a non pathogenic rabbit haemorrhagic disease-like virus. *Veterinary Record*, 140, 647–50.

Carpenter, J.W., Mashima, T.Y. & Rupiper, D.J. (2001) Rabbits. In: *Exotic Animal Formulary* (2nd Edn). W.B. Saunders, Philadelphia, pp. 300–26.

Catchpole, J. & Norton, C.C. (1979) The species of *Eimeria* in rabbits for meat production in Britain. *Parasitology*, 79, 249–57.

Chasey, D. (1997) Rabbit haemorrhagic disease, the new scourge of *Oryctolagus cuniculus*. *Laboratory Animals*, 31, 33–44.

Chasey, D., Lucas, M.H., Westcott, D.G., Sharp, G., Kitching, A. & Hughes, S.K. (1995) Development of a diagnostic approach to the identification of rabbit haemorrhagic disease. *Veterinary Record*, 137, 158–60.

Clampitt, R.B. & Hart, R.J. (1978) The tissue activities of some diagnostic enzymes in ten mammalian species. *Journal of Comparative Pathology*, 88, 607–21.

Clard, J.D., Jain, A.V. & Hatch, R.C. (1980) Experimentally induced chronic aflatoxicosis in rabbits. *American Journal of Veterinary Research*, 41, 1841–5.

Clippinger, T.L., Bennet, R.A., Alleman, A.R., Ginn, P.E. & Bellah, J.R. (1998) Removal of a thymoma via median sternotomy in a rabbit with recurrent appendicular neurofibrosarcoma. *Journal of the American Veterinary Medical Association*, 213(8), 1140–3.

Coke, R. (2002) Surgical removal of a urolith from a rabbit's distal urethra. *Veterinary Medicine*, 97, 514–8.

Cooke, S.W. (2000) Clinical chemistry. In: Flecknell, P. (Ed.), *BSAVA Manual of Rabbit Medicine and Surgery*. British Small Animal Veterinary Association, Quedgeley, pp. 25–32.

Crossley, D.A. (1994) Extraction of rabbit incisor teeth. *Proceedings of the European Veterinary Dental Society Forum 1994*.

Crossley, D.A. (1995) Clinical aspects of lagomorph dental anatomy: the rabbit (*Oryctolagus cuniculus*). *Journal of Veterinary Dentistry*, 12, 137–40.

Crossley, D.A. (2000) Diagnosis of dental disease in rabbits and rodents. In: *Proceedings of the North American Veterinary Conference*, pp. 993–4.

Curiel, T.J., Perfect, J.R. & Durack, D.T. (1982) Leukocyte subpopulations in cerebrospinal fluid of normal rabbits. *Laboratory Animal Science*, 32, 622.

Davies, O. (2004) Diseases of the growing rabbit. In: Meredith, A. (Ed.), *CD-Lapis*. Vetstream, Winchester.

Davies, O. (2004) Hereditary conditions. In: Meredith, A. (Ed.), *CD-Lapis*. Vetstream, Winchester.

Dawson, S. & Meredith, A. (2004) Papilloma virus. In: Meredith, A. (Ed.), *CD-Lapis*. Vetstream, Winchester.

Deeb, B.J. (1997) Respiratory disease and the Pasteurella complex. In: Hillyer, E.V. & Quesenberry, K.E. (Eds) *Ferrets, Rabbits and Rodents: Clinical Medicine and Surgery*. W.B. Saunders, Philadelphia, pp. 189–201.

Deeb, B. (2000) Digestive system and disorders. In: Flecknell, P. (Ed.), *BSAVA Manual of Rabbit Medicine and Surgery*. British Small Animal Veterinary Association, Quedgeley, pp. 39–46.

Deeb, B.J. & Carpenter, J.W. (2004) Neurological and musculoskeletal diseases. In: Quesenberry, K.E. & Carpenter, J.W. (Eds), *Ferrets, Rabbits and Rodents: Clinical Medicine and Surgery* (2nd Edn). W.B. Saunders, Philadelphia, pp. 203–10.

Deeb, B.J. & DiGiacomo, R.F. (2000) Respiratory diseases of rabbits. *Veterinary Clinics of North America Exotic Animal Practice*, 3(2), 465–80.

Deeb, B.J., DiGiacomo, R.F., Bernard, B.L. & Silbernagel, S.M. (1990) *Pasteurella multocida* and *Bordetella bronchiseptica* infections in rabbits. *Journal of Clinical Microbiology*, 28, 70–75.

Deplazes, P., Mathis, A., Baumgartner, R., Tanner, I. & Weber, R. (1996) Immunologic and molecular characteristics of *Encephalitozoon*-like microsporidia isolated from humans and rabbits indicate that *Encephalitozoon cuniculi* is a zoonotic parasite. *Clinical Infectious Diseases*, 22(3), 557–9.

DiGiacomo, R.F. & Mare, C.J. (1994) Viral diseases. In: Manning, P.J., Ringler, D.H.
    & Newcomer, C.E. (Eds), *The Biology of the Laboratory Rabbit* (2nd Edn).
    Academic Press, San Diego, pp. 171–204.

DiGiacomo, R.F., Talburt, C.D., Lukehart, S.A., Baker-Zander, S.A., Condon, J. (1983)
    Treponema paraluis cuniculi infection in a commercial rabbitry: epidemiology and
    serodiagnosis. *Laboratory Animal Science*, 33, 562–6.

Divers, S.J. & Lafortune, M. (2000) Rabbit dyspnoea, rabbit rhinitis, rabbit pneumonia.
    In: Meredith, A. (Ed.), *CD-Lapis*. Vetstream, Winchester.

Divers, S.J. & Lafortune, M. (2000) Investigating dyspnoea in the rabbit. *Veterinary
    Times*, 30(3), 10.

Divers, S.J. & Mitchell, M. (2000) Endoscopic evaluation of lagomorphs. In:
    Proceedings of the European Association of Zoo and Wildlife Veterinarians Meeting,
    Paris, pp. 221–6.

Dodds, W.J. (2000) Disorders of rabbit and ferret haemostasis. In: Fudge, A.M. (Ed.),
    Laboratory Medicine: Avian and Exotic Pets. W.B. Saunders, Philadelphia,
    pp. 285–90.

Donnelly, T.M. (2004) Basic anatomy, physiology and husbandry. In: Quesenberry,
    K.E. & Carpenter, J.W. (Eds), *Ferrets, Rabbits and Rodents: Clinical Medicine and
    Surgery* (2nd Edn). W.B. Saunders, Philadelphia, pp. 136–46.

Dykes, L. (2003) Sticky bums: understanding caecotrophy. *Rabbiting On*, Summer.
    Rabbit Welfare Association, Horsham.

Dykes, L. (2004) Nutritional support for convalescing rabbits. *Veterinary Nurse Times*,
    July, pp. 8–10.

Easson, W. (2001) A review of rabbit and rodent production medicine. *Seminars in
    Avian and Exotic Pet Medicine*, 10, 131–9.

Ellis, T.M., Gregory, A.R., Logue, G.D. (1991) Evaluation of a toxoid for protection
    of rabbits against enterotoxaemia experimentally induced by trypsin-activated
    supernatant of *Clostridium spiroforme*. *Veterinary Microbiology*, 28, 93–102.

Emily, P. (1991) Problems peculiar to continually erupting teeth. *Journal of Small
    Animal Exotic Medicine*, 1, 56–9.

Evering, W. & Edwards, J.F. (1992) Hepatic lobe deformity in a rabbit. *Laboratory
    Animals*, 21, 14–16.

Fairham, J. & Harcourt-Brown, F.M. (1999) Preliminary investigation of the vitamin D
    status of pet rabbits. *Veterinary Record*, 145, 452–4.

Feaga, W.P. (1997) Wry neck in rabbits. *Journal of the American Veterinary Medical
    Association*, 210(4), 480.

Fenner, F. & Fantani, B. (1999) *Biological Control of Vertebrate Pests: The History of
    Myxomatosis – An Experiment in Evolution*. CABI Publishing, Wallingford.

Fenner, F. & Ross, J. (1994) Myxomatosis. In: Thompson, H.V. & King, C.M. (Eds),
    The European Rabbit: The History and Biology of a Successful Colonizer. Oxford
    University Press, Oxford, pp. 205–35.

Flecknell, P. (1998) Developments in the veterinary care of rabbits and rodents. *In
    Practice*, 20, 6.

Fox, R.R., Meier, H., Crary, D.D., Norberg, R.F. & Myers, D.D. (1971) Hemolytic
    anemia associated with thymoma in the rabbit. Genetic studies and pathological
    findings. *Oncology*, 25(4), 372–82.

Fudge, A.M. (2000) Rabbit hematology. In: Fudge, A.M. (Ed.), *Laboratory Medicine: Avian and Exotic Pets*. W.B. Saunders, Philadelphia, pp. 273–5.

Garcia del Blanco, N., Gutierrez, C.B., de la Puente, V.A. & Rodriguez Ferri, E.F. (2004) Biochemical characterisation of *Francisella tularensis* strains isolated in Spain. *Veterinary Record*, 154, 55–6.

Gentz, E.J. & Carpenter, J.W. (1997) Rabbits: neurologic and musculoskeletal disease. In: Hillyer E.V. & Quesenberry K.E. (Eds), *Ferrets, Rabbits and Rodents: Clinical Medicine and Surgery*. W.B. Saunders, Philadelphia, pp. 220–6.

Gillett, N.A., Brooks, D.L. & Tillman, P.C. (1983) Medical and surgical management of gastric obstruction from a hairball in the rabbit. *Journal of the American Veterinary Medical Association*, 183(11), 1176–8.

Girling, S. (2003) Small mammal nutrition. In: *Veterinary Nursing of Exotic Pets*. Blackwell, Oxford, pp. 246–56.

Glavits, R. & Magyar, T. (1990) The pathology of experimental respiratory infection with *Pasteurella multocida* and *Bordetella bronchiseptica* in rabbits. *Acta Veterinaria Hungarica*, 38, 211–5.

Gobel, T. (2002) Transurethral uroendoscopy in the female rabbit. *Exotic DVM*, 4(5), 23–7.

Gomez, L., Gazquez, A., Roncero, V., Sanchez, C. & Duran, M.E. (2002) Lymphoma in a rabbit: histopathological and immunohistochemical findings. *Journal of Small Animal Practice*, 43(5), 224–6.

Grest, P., Albicker, P., Hoelzle, L., Wild, P. & Pospischil, A. (2002) Herpes simplex encephalitis in a domestic rabbit (*Oryctolagus cuniculus*). *Journal of Comparative Pathology*, 126(4), 308–11.

Gustafsson, K., Wattrang, E., Fossum, C., Heegaard, P.M., Lind, P. & Uggla, A. (1997) *Toxoplasma gondii* infection in the mountain hare (*Lepus timidus*) and the domestic rabbit (*Oryctolagus cuniculus*). Parts I and II. *Journal of Comparative Pathology*, 117(4), 351–69.

Harcourt-Brown, F. (1996) Calcium deficiency, diet and dental disease in pet rabbits. *Veterinary. Record*, 139, 567–71.

Harcourt-Brown, F. (1997) Diagnosis, treatment and prognosis of dental disease in pet rabbits. *In Practice*, 18, 407–21.

Harcourt-Brown, F. (2002) *Textbook of Rabbit Medicine*. Butterworth-Heinemann, Oxford.

Harcourt-Brown, F. (2002) Update on metabolic bone disease in rabbits. *Exotic DVM*, 4(3), 43–6.

Harcourt-Brown, F. (2002) Intestinal obstruction in rabbits. *Exotic DVM*, 4(3), 51–3.

Harcourt-Brown, F. (2002) Anorexia in rabbits 1. Causes and effects. *In Practice*, 24(7), 358–67.

Harcourt-Brown, F. (2002) Anorexia in rabbits 2. Diagnosis and treatment. *In Practice*, 24(8), 450–67.

Harcourt-Brown, F. (2004) Calcium metabolism in rabbits. *Exotic DVM*, 6(2), 11–14.

Harcourt-Brown, F. (2004) *Encephalitozoon cuniculi* infection in rabbits. *Seminars in Avian and Exotic Pet Medicine*, 13(2), 86–93.

Harcourt Brown, F. (2004) Sudden death in pet rabbits. *Rabbiting On*, Summer, p. 7, Horsham.

Harcourt-Brown, F.M. & Holloway, H.K. (2003) *Encephalitozoon cuniculi* in pet
    rabbits. *Veterinary Record*, **152**(14), 427–31.
Hernandez-Divers, S.J. & Murray, M. (2004) Small mammal endoscopy. In:
    Quesenberry, K.E. & Carpenter, J.W. (Eds), *Ferrets, Rabbits and Rodents:
    Clinical Medicine and Surgery* (2nd Edn). W.B. Saunders, Philadelphia, pp. 392–4.
Hess, L. (2004) Dermatologic diseases. In: Quesenberry, K.E. & Carpenter, J.W. (Eds),
    Ferrets, Rabbits and Rodents: Clinical Medicine and Surgery (2nd Edn). W.B.
    Saunders, Philadelphia, pp. 194–202.
Hillyer, E.V. (1994) Pet rabbits. *Veterinary Clinics of North America Small Animal
    Practice*, **24**(1), 25–65.
Hoefer, H.L. (2000) Rabbit and ferret renal disease diagnosis. In: Fudge, A.M. (Ed.),
    Laboratory Medicine: Avian and Exotic Pets. W.B. Saunders, Philadelphia, pp.
    311–8.
Hohenboken, W.D. & Nellhaus, G. (1970) Inheritance of audiogenic seizures in the
    rabbit. *Journal of Heredity*, **61**(3), 107–12.
Holloway, H.K.R. & Carmichael, N.G. (2001) Significance of serum fructosamine in
    rabbits. *Proceedings of the British Small Animal Veterinary Association Congress*,
    p. 554.
Hugget, C. (2004) Poisonous plants. *Rabbiting On*, Spring. Rabbit Welfare Association,
    Horsham.
Hugget, C. (2004) Feeding the convalescent rabbit. *Rabbiting On*, Autumn. Rabbit
    Welfare Association, Horsham.
Huston, S.M. & Quesenberry, K.E. (2004) Cardiovascular and hemopoetic diseases.
    In: Quesenberry, K.E. & Carpenter, J.W. (Eds), *Ferrets, Rabbits and Rodents:
    Clinical Medicine and Surgery* (2nd Edn), W.B. Saunders, Philadelphia,
    pp. 211–20.
Ikaheimo, I., Syrjala, H., Karhukorpi, J., Schildt, R. & Koskela, M. (2000) *In vitro*
    antibiotic susceptibility of *Francisella tularensis* isolated from humans and animals.
    Journal of Antimicrobial Chemotherapy, **46**(2), 287–90.
Jackson, G. (1991) Intestinal stasis and rupture in rabbits. *Veterinary Record*,
    129(13), 287–9.
Jenkins, J.R. (1997) Gastrointestinal diseases. In: Hillyer, E.V. and Quesenberry, K.E.
    (Eds) *Ferrets, Rabbits and Rodents: Clinical Medicine and Surgery*. W.B. Saunders,
    London.
Jenkins, J.R. (2000) Rabbit and ferret liver and gastrointestinal testing. In: Fudge, A.M.
    (Ed.), *Laboratory Medicine: Avian and Exotic Pets*. W.B. Saunders, Philadelphia,
    pp. 291–304.
Jenkins, J.R. (2003) Rabbit behavior. *Veterinary Clinics of North America Exotic
    Animal Practice*, **4**(3), 669–79.
Jenkins, J.R. (2004a) Gastrointestinal diseases. In: Quesenberry, K.E. & Carpenter,
    J.W. (Eds), *Ferrets, Rabbits and Rodents: Clinical Medicine and Surgery* (2nd Edn).
    W.B. Saunders, Philadelphia, pp. 161–71.
Jenkins, J.R. (2004b) Soft tissue surgery. In: Quesenberry, K.E. & Carpenter, J.W.
    (Eds), *Ferrets, Rabbits and Rodents: Clinical Medicine and Surgery*. W.B. Saunders,
    Philadelphia, pp. 221–31.
Jones, J.R. & Duff, J.P. (2001) Rabbit epizootic enterocolitis (letter). *Veterinary Record*,
    149(17), 532.

Joyner, L.P., Catchpole, J. & Berret, S. (1983) *Eimeria stiedai* in rabbits: the demonstration of different responses to chemotherapy. *Research in Veterinary Science*, 34, 64–7.

Keeble, E. (2001) Endocrine diseases in small mammals. *In Practice*, 23(10), 570–85.

Kostolich, M. & Panciera, R.J. (1992) Thymoma in a rabbit. *Cornell Veterinarian*, 82(2), 125–9.

Kunstyr, I. & Naumann, S. (1985) Head tilt in rabbits caused by pasteurellosis and encephalitozoonosis. *Laboratory Animals*, 19, 208–13.

Kunstyr, I., Lev, L. & Naumann, S. (1986) Humoral antibody response to experimental infection with *Encephalitozoon cuniculi*. *Veterinary Parasitology*, 21, 223–32.

Kusumi, R.K. & Plouffe, J.F. (1980) Cerebrospinal fluid glucose and protein values in normal rabbits. *Laboratory Animals*, 14, 41–2.

Lang, J. (1981) The nutrition of the commercial rabbit. Part 1. Physiology, digestibility and nutrient requirements. *Nutrition Abstracts Review Series B*, 51, 197–217.

Lee, K.J., Johnson, W.D., Lang, C.M. & Hartshorn, R.D. (1978) Hydronephrosis caused by urinary lithiasis in a New Zealand White rabbit (*Oryctolagus cuniculus*). *Veterinary Pathology*, 15(5), 676–8.

Leland, M.L., Hubbard, G.B. & Dubey, J.P. (1992) Clinical toxoplasmosis in domestic rabbits. *Laboratory Animal Science*, 42(3), 318–9.

Lindsey, J.R. & Fox, R.R. (1994) Inherited diseases and variations. In: Manning, P.J., Ringler, D.H. & Newcomer, C.E. (Eds), *The Biology of the Laboratory Rabbit* (2nd Edn). Academic Press, New York, pp. 293–319.

Lipman, N.S., Zhi-Bo, Z., Andrutis, K.A., Hurley, R.J., Fox, J.G. & White, H.J. (1994) Prolactin secreting pituitary adenomas with mammary dysplasia in New Zealand White rabbits. *Laboratory Animal Science*, 44, 114–20.

Lobprise, H.B. & Wiggs, R.B. (1991) Dental diseases in lagomorphs. *Journal of Veterinary Dentistry*, 8, 11–17.

Longley, L. (2004) Supportive care of rabbits. *Veterinary Times*, 1st March.

Loutsch, J.M., Sainz, B., Jr, Marquart, M.E., Zheng, X., Kesavan, P., Higaki, S., Hill, J.M. & Tal-Singer, R. (2001) Effect of famciclovir on herpes simplex virus type 1 corneal disease and establishment of latency in rabbits. *Antimicrobial Agents and Chemotherapy*, 45(7), 2044–53.

Mader, D.R. (1997) Rabbits: basic approach to veterinary care. In: Hillyer, E.V. & Quesenberry, K.E. (Eds), *Ferrets, Rabbits and Rodents: Clinical Medicine and Surgery*. W.B. Saunders, Philadelphia, pp. 160–8.

Makkar, H.P.S. & Singh, B. (1991) Aflatoxicosis in rabbits. *Journal of Applied Rabbit Research*, 14, 218–22.

Malley, A.D. (2000) Handling, restraint and clinical techniques. In: Flecknell, P. (Ed.), *BSAVA Manual of Rabbit Medicine and Surgery*. British Small Animal Veterinary Association, Quedgeley, pp. 1–12.

Meredith, A. (2000) General biology and husbandry. In: Flecknell, P. (Ed.), *BSAVA Manual of Rabbit Medicine and Surgery*. British Small Animal Veterinary Association, Quedgeley, pp. 13–23.

Meredith, A. (2004) Liver disease in the rabbit. *Veterinary Times*, 1st March, pp. 14–15.

Meredith, A. (2004) (Ed.) *CD-Lapis*. Vetstream, Winchester.

Meredith, A. & O'Malley, B. (2004) Spinal injury. In: Meredith, A. (Ed.), *CD-Lapis*. Vetstream, Winchester.

Morgan, R.V., Moore, F.M., Pearce, L.K. & Rossi, T. (1991) Clinical and laboratory findings in small companion animals with lead poisoning: 347 cases (1977–1986). *Journal of the American Veterinary Medical Association*, **199**(1), 93–7.

Munoz, M.E., Gonzales, J. & Esteller, A. (1986) Bile pigment formation and excretion in the rabbit. *Comparative Biochemistry and Physiology Part A*, **85**, 67–71.

Murray, M.J. (2000) Rabbit and ferret sampling and artefact considerations. In: Fudge, A.M. (Ed.), *Laboratory Medicine: Avian and Exotic Pets*. W.B. Saunders, Philadelphia, pp. 265–8.

Ness, R.D. (1998) Neoplasia in rabbits and guinea pigs. *Proceedings of the North American Veterinary Conference*, pp. 853–4.

Okerman, L. (1994) *Diseases of Domestic Rabbits* (2nd Edn). Blackwell, Oxford.

Okerman, L., Devriese, L.A., Gevaert, D., Uyttebroek, D. & Haesebrouck, F. (1990) *In vivo* activity of orally administered antibiotics and chemotherapeutics against acute septicaemic pasteurellosis in rabbits. *Laboratory Animals*, **24**, 341–4.

Onderka, D.K., Papp-Vid, G. & Perry, A.W. (1992) Fatal herpes virus infection in commercial rabbits. *Canadian Veterinary Journal*, **33**, 539–43.

Orcutt, C. (2000) Parenteral nutrition for small exotic herbivores. *Exotic DVM*, **2**(3), 39–43.

Orcutt, C. (2000) Use of oxyglobin in exotic animals. In: *Proceedings of the British Veterinary Zoological Society Autumn Meeting: Critical Care and Emergency Medicine*, pp. 61–3.

Owen D.G. & Gannon, J. (1980) Investigation into the trans-placental transmission of *Encephalitozoon cuniculi* in rabbits. *Laboratory Animals*, **14**, 35–8.

Pakes, S.P. & Gerrity, L.W. (1994) Protozoal diseases. In: Manning, P.J., Ringler, D.H. & Newcomer, C.E. (Eds) *The Biology of the Laboratory Rabbit* (2nd Edn). Academic Press, San Diego, p. 206.

Pare, J.A. & Paul-Murphy, J. (2004) Disorders of the reproductive and urinary systems. In: Quesenberry, K.E. & Carpenter, J.W. (Eds), *Ferrets, Rabbits and Rodents: Clinical Medicine and Surgery*. W.B. Saunders, Philadelphia, pp. 183–93.

Patton, S. (2000) Rabbit and ferret parasite testing. In: Fudge, A.M. (Ed.), *Laboratory Medicine: Avian and Exotic Pets*. W.B. Saunders, Philadelphia, pp. 358–66.

Paul-Murphy, J. & Ramer, J. (1998) Urgent care of the pet rabbit. *Veterinary Clinics of North America Exotic Animal Practice*, **1**(1), 127–52.

Peeters, J.E. & Geeroms, R. (1986) Efficacy of toltrazuril against intestinal and hepatic coccidiosis of rabbits. *Veterinary Parasitology*, **1**, 21–35.

Potter, M.P. & Borkowski, G.L. (1998) Apparent psychogenic polydipsia and secondary polyuria in laboratory housed New Zealand White rabbits. *Contemporary Topics*, **37**, 87–9.

Raftery, A. (2001) Occult blood testing in rabbits. *Proceedings of the British Veterinary Zoological Society Meeting*, p. 53.

Reavill, D.R. & Schmidt, R.E. (2000) Rabbit surgical pathology. In: Fudge, A.M. (Ed.), *Laboratory Medicine: Avian and Exotic Pets*. W.B. Saunders, Philadelphia, pp. 353–66.

Redrobe, S. (2000) Surgical procedures and dental disorders. In: Flecknell, P. (Ed.), *BSAVA Manual of Rabbit Medicine and Surgery*. British Small Animal Veterinary Association, Quedgeley, pp. 117–34.

Redrobe, S. (2000) Urogenital system and disorders. In: Flecknell, P. (Ed.), *BSAVA Manual of Rabbit Medicine and Surgery*. British Small Animal Veterinary Association, Quedgeley, pp. 47–55.

Rees Davies, R. & Rees Davies, J.A.E. (2003) Rabbit gastrointestinal physiology. *Veterinary Clinics of North America Exotic Animal Practice*, 6, 139–53.

Richardson, V.C.G. (2000) *Rabbits: Health, Husbandry and Disease*. Blackwell Science, Oxford.

Richardson, V. (2003) *Russel and Gerty's Guide to Dangerous Plants*. Supreme Petfoods, Hants.

Rogers, G., Taylor, C., Austin, J.C. & Rosen, C. (1988) A pharyngostomy technique for chronic oral dosing of rabbits. *Laboratory Animal Science*, 38, 619–20.

Rosenthal, K.L. (2000) Ferret and rabbit endocrine disease diagnosis. In: Fudge, A.M. (Ed.), *Laboratory Medicine: Avian and Exotic Pets*. W.B. Saunders, Philadelphia, pp. 319–24.

Roth, S. & Conway, H. (1982) Animal model of human disease. Spontaneous diabetes mellitus in the New Zealand White rabbit. *American Journal of Pathology*, 109, 359–63.

Rutgers, H.C. (1994) The alimentary system. In: Chandler, E.A., Gaskell, C.J. & Gaskell, R.M. (Eds), *Feline Medicine and Therapeutics* (2nd Edn). Blackwell Scientific, Oxford, pp. 287–321.

Salama, M.N., Tsuji, M., Tamura, M. & Kagawa, S. (1998) Immediate effects of extracorporeal shock waves on the male genital system of rabbits. Preliminary report. *Scandinavian Journal of Urology and Nephrology*, 32(4), 251–5.

Samman, S., Fussell, S.H. & Rose, C.I. (1991) Porphyria in a New Zealand White rabbit. *Canadian Veterinary Journal*, 32, 622–3.

Schmidt, R.E. (1995) Protozoal diseases of rabbits and rodents. *Seminars in Avian and Exotic Pet Medicine*, 4, 126–30.

Schoenbaum, M. & Kapeller, S. (1982) Three apparent cases of tetanus in rabbits. *Refuah Veterinarith*, 39(1/2), 15–16.

Shell, L.G. & Saunders, G. (1989) Arteriosclerosis in a rabbit. *Journal of the American Veterinary Medical Association*, 194, 679–80.

Shibuya, K., Tajima, M., Kanai, K., Ihara, M. & Nunoya, T. (1999) Spontaneous lymphoma in a Japanese White rabbit. *Journal of Veterinary Medical Science*, 61(12), 1327–9.

Smith, D.A., Olson, P.O. & Matthews, K.A. (1997) Nutritional support for rabbits using the percutaneously placed gastrostomy tube: a preliminary study. *Journal of the American Animal Hospital Association*, 33(1), 48–54.

Stiles, J., Didier, E., Ritchie, B., Greenacre, C., Willis, M. & Martin, C. (1997) *Encephalitozoon cuniculi* in the lens of a rabbit with phacoclastic uveitis: confirmation and treatment. *Veterinary Comparative Ophthalmology*, 7, 233–8.

Sturgess, K. (2003) *Notes on Feline Internal Medicine*. Blackwell Publishing, Oxford.

Suter, C., Muller-Doblies, U.U., Hatt, J.-M. & Deplazes, P. (2001) Prevention and treatment of *Encephalitozoon cuniculi* in rabbits with fenbendazole. *Veterinary Record*, 148, 478–80.

Swartout, M.S. & Gerken, D.F. (1987) Lead induced toxicosis in two domestic rabbits. *Journal of the American Veterinary Medical Association*, 197, 717–19.

Tosic, M., Dolivo, M., Amiguet, P., Domanska-Janik, K. & Matthieu, J.M. (1993)
Paralytic tremor (pt) rabbit: a sex-linked mutation affecting proteolipid protein-gene
expression. *Brain Research*, **625**(2), 307–12.

Van Kampen, K.R. (1968) Lymphosarcoma in the rabbit. A case report and general
review. *Cornell Veterinarian*, **58**(1), 121–8.

Various (2004) *Behavior.* House Rabbit Society. (http://www.rabbit.org/ behavior/
index.html) Accessed 12/11/2004.

Vernau, K.M., Grahn, B.H., Clarke-Scott, H.A. & Sullivan, N. (1995) Thymoma in a
geriatric rabbit with hypercalcaemia and periodic exophthalmos. *Journal of the
American Veterinary Medical Association*, **206**(11), 1675–7.

Verstraete, F.J.M. (2003) Advances in diagnosis and treatment of small exotic
mammal dental disease. *Seminars in Avian and Exotic Pet Medicine*, **12**(1),
37–48.

Vistelle, R., Jaussaud, R., Trenque, T. & Wiczewski, M. (1994) Rapid and simple
cannulation technique for repeated sampling of cerebrospinal fluid in the conscious
rabbit. *Laboratory Animal Science*, **44**(4), 362–4.

Warns, E. (1997) Encephalitozoonosis: a possible treatment for rabbits? *Lapin Lines*,
4(4), 1–7.

Waters, M. (2004) Blood biochemistry: ALT, AST, ALP. In: Meredith, A. (Ed.),
CD-Lapis. Vetstream, Winchester.

Waters, M. (2004) Blood biochemistry: sodium, chloride, calcium, potassium,
phosphate. In: Meredith, A. (Ed.), *CD-Lapis*. Vetstream, Winchester.

Waters, M. (2004) Blood biochemistry: total protein, albumin, globulin. In: Meredith,
A. (Ed.), *CD-Lapis*. Vetstream, Winchester.

Waters, M. (2004) Blood biochemistry: urea and creatinine. In: Meredith, A. (Ed.),
CD-Lapis. Vetstream, Winchester.

Waters, M. (2004) Haematology: basophil, eosinophil, leukocyte, lymphocyte,
neutrophil. In: Meredith, A. (Ed.), *CD-Lapis*. Vetstream, Winchester.

Waters, M. (2004) Haematology: nucleated red blood cells. In: Meredith, A. (Ed.),
CD-Lapis. Vetstream, Winchester.

Waters, M. (2004) Urinalysis: dipstick analysis. In: Meredith, A. (Ed.), *CD-Lapis*.
Vetstream, Winchester.

Watson, L.C. & Blackburn, C.R. (1956) The pressure and calcium concentration of the
cerebrospinal fluid of the rabbit. *Australian Journal of Experimental Biology and
Medical Science*, **34**(1), 53–8.

Watson, W.T., Goldsboro, J.A., Williams, F.P. & Sueur, R. (1975) Experimental
respiratory infection with *Pasteurella multocida* and *Bordetella bronchiseptica* in
rabbits. *Laboratory Animal Science*, **25**, 459–64.

Weisbroth, S.H. (1994) Neoplastic diseases. In: Manning, P.J., Ringler, D.H. &
Newcomer C.E. (Eds), *The Biology of the Laboratory Rabbit*
(2nd Edn). Academic Press, New York, pp. 259–92.

Weisbroth, S.H., Flatt, R.E. & Kraus, A.L. (Eds) (1974) Values for constituents of
rabbit cerebrospinal fluid. In: *The Biology of the Laboratory Rabbit*. Academic Press,
New York, p. 65.

Weissenbock, H., Hainfellner, J.A., Berger, J., Kasper, I. & Budka, H. (1977) Naturally
occurring herpes simplex encephalitis in a domestic rabbit (*Oryctolagus cuniculus*).
Veterinary Pathology, **34**, 44–7.

White, R.N. (2001) Management of calcium ureterolithiasis in a French Lop rabbit. *Journal of Small Animal Practice*, **42**, 595–8.

White, R.N. (2004) CT scan of liver cyst. In: Meredith, A. (Ed.), *CD-Lapis*. Vetstream, Winchester.

Wiggs, B. & Lobprise, H. (1995) Dental anatomy and physiology of pet rodents and lagomorphs. In: Crossley, D.A. & Penman, S. (Eds), *BSAVA Manual of Small Animal Dentistry* (2nd Edn). British Small Animal Veterinary Association, Cheltenham, pp. 68–73.

Wiggs, B. & Lobprise, H. (1995) Oral diagnosis in pet rodents and lagomorphs. In: Crossley, D.A. & Penman, S. (Eds), *BSAVA Manual of Small Animal Dentistry* (2nd Edn). British Small Animal Veterinary Association, Cheltenham, pp. 74–83.

Wiggs, B & Lobprise, H. (1995) Prevention and treatment of dental problems in rodents and lagomorphs. In: Crossley, D.A. & Penman, S. (Eds), *BSAVA Manual of Small Animal Dentistry* (2nd Edn). British Small Animal Veterinary Association, Cheltenham, pp. 84–91.

Williams, B.H. (2000) Disorders of rabbit and ferret bone marrow. In: Fudge, A.M. (Ed.), *Laboratory Medicine: Avian and Exotic Pets*. W.B. Saunders, Philadelphia, pp. 276–84.

Yamini, B. & Stein, S. (1989) Abortion, stillbirth, neonatal death and nutritional myodegeneration in a rabbit breeding colony. *Journal of the American Veterinary Medical Association*, **194**, 561–2.

Yousef, M.I., El-Demerdash, F.M. & Al-Salhen, K.S. (2003) Protective role of isoflavones against the toxic effect of cypermethrin on semen quality and testosterone levels of rabbits. *Journal of Environmental Science and Health Series B*, **38**(4), 463–78.

Zwicker, G.M., Killinger, J.M. & McConnel, R.F. (1985) Spontaneous vesicular and prostatic gland epithelial squamous metaplasia, hyperplasia, and keratinized nodule formation in rabbits. *Toxicologic Pathology*, **13**(3), 222–8.

INDEX

abdominal distension, 3, 15, 92, 135
abdominal enlargement, 27, 128, 133, 138, 142, 147, 168, 170
abdominal pain, 6, 13, 34, 50, 127, 128, 133–4
abdominocentesis, 8–10
abortion, 43–5, 106, 137, 168, 187
abscess, 3–4, 49, 72, 98, 119–24, 128, 191
ACE inhibitors, 93
acidosis, 28, 77, 157
acute renal failure, 156
acquired dental disease, 6, 118–20
adhesions, 4, 133, 139, 206
aflatoxin, 47, 67, 79, 81, 142, 145
air fresheners, 61, 95, 190
alfalfa, 37, 114
ammonia, 28, 61, 80, 95–6, 190
amyloid, 83, 158
anabolic steroids, 157, 159, 207
anaemia, 16, 27, 63, 71–3, 107, 158
anaerobes, 98, 121, 191, 202–3
anorexia, 6, 46, 67, 79, 84, 104, 110, 119, 122, 126–8, 133, 140, 142, 144, 181
antibiotic related diarrhoea/enterotoxaemia, 21, 134, 140–41, 202
anticoagulant rodenticide, 13, 37–9, 173
aortic mineralization, 15, 91, 106, 154
appetite stimulants, 129
arteriosclerosis, 91–2, 186
ascarid, 60, 103, 186
ascites, 8, 20, 99, 128, 133, 142–4, 181–2
aspartate aminotransferase (AST), 80
aspiration pneumonia, 18, 111
ataxia, 11, 103–5, 184
atherosclerosis, 14–15, 51, 91–2, 108
atopy, 74
atrophic rhinitis, 28
aural disease, 56
azotaemia, 75–6, 85, 150, 156–8

Baylisascaris procyonis, 41, 102, 186
behaviour, 12, 46, 53, 55, 101, 172, 184
benzodiazepines, 7, 94, 161, 205
bile, 8, 11, 78
bile acids, 80, 144, 182
bilirubin/biliverdin, 46, 81, 182
bladder, 4, 9, 38, 75, 77, 83, 159–65

bleeding disorder, 13, 35, 38–40, 72, 173
blowflies, *see* myiasis
Bordatella bronchiseptica, 28, 40, 61, 95–6, 102, 177, 190–91, 201
botulism, 26, 56, 103
bronchoalveolar lavage, 19, 29, 96–7
bronchopneumonia, 18, 28, 96, 188–90

caecal dysbiosis, 108, 140
caecal impaction/dilation, 4, 6, 140
caecotroph, 6, 13, 32, 35, 51, 85–6, 107, 133–5
caecotroph accumulation, 13, 19, 26, 50–51, 85, 97, 115, 133–5, 165
caecum, 32, 133, 140
cagemate (loss of), 6, 33
calcium, 76–7, 91, 106, 114, 152, 159
calcium oxalate, 152, 160–63
calculi (cystic/urinary), 9, 33, 37, 152, 160
calicivirus (VHD), 16, 22, 35, 37–8, 47, 60, 63–4, 67, 81, 96, 98, 147–8, 173, 177–9, 186
campylobacter, 22, 86, 137
carbon monoxide, 12, 27
cardiac disease, 14–16, 27, 63, 67–8, 75, 91–3, 96, 99, 184
cardiomyopathy, 15, 63, 91, 184
castration, 45, 165
cataract, 184
cereal based diet, 19, 51, 108
cerebellar hypoplasia, 11
cerebrospinal fluid, 87–8
cerebrovascular emboli, 41, 60, 91, 102, 178, 186
Cheyletiella, 188
cholestasis, 46
cholesterol, 71, 78, 144, 149
cholestyramine, 141, 206
chronic renal failure, 188–9
chyle, 8, 11, 98
circling, 12, 103, 186
cisapride, 130, 206
clagging, *see* caecotroph accumulation
clay, 32
Clostridium, 132, 140–41
Clostridium piliforme, 21, 87, 137, 146, 196
Clostridium spiroforme, 21, 87, 113, 141